The
Pocket
Herbal

REFERENCE

2nd Edition

Rita Elkins, M.H.
Author of *Solving the Depression Puzzle*

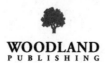

WOODLAND
PUBLISHING

For ordering information, contact:
Woodland Publishing, P.O. Box 160, Pleasant Grove, Utah 84062
(800) 777-2665

Note: The information in this book is for educational purposes only and is not
recommended as a means of diagnosing or treating an illness. All matters concerning physical and mental health should be supervised by a health practitioner
knowledgeable in treating that particular condition. Neither the publisher nor
author directly or indirectly dispenses medical advice, nor do they prescribe any
remedies or assume any responsibility for those who choose to treat themselves.

A CIP record for this book is available from the Library of Congress.

ISBN 1-58054-099-6

Second Edition

10 9 8 7 6 5 4 3 2 1

Printed in the United States of America

Please visit our website:
www.woodlandpublishing.com

Contents

Introduction

Fifteen years ago I scoffed at the use of vitamins, minerals and herbs. Today, after years of research, I write and lecture about their value with great enthusiasm. Now, more than ever before, having reliable information about the enormous number of dietary supplements that surround us is crucial. In designing this ready reference, I used my own personal wish list for a information-at-my-fingertip guide to natural health compounds. I wanted the following features:

- Information that leads to the selection of best supplements for individual needs
- Therapeutic applications for individual herbs, vitamins, etc.
- Product familiarity: is it potent, what does it do, is it safe?

It's estimated that up to 100 million North Americans routinely take dietary supplements. But have they chosen wisely? Interestingly, statistics tell us that supplement takers tend to be more educated, more affluent, and more healthy. If you want to join the ranks of those who use nutritional supplements, you need easy-access to facts to make wise purchases. Walking through the supplement aisles of a health food store can be mind boggling to say the least. A hands-on-guide is an absolute necessity. This pocket reference supplies you with a concise overview of the six most important kinds of supplements:

- vitamins and minerals
- herbs
- phytonutrients
- hormones
- amino acids and antioxidants
- other natural compounds

The "other" refers to supplements that don't fit the category of either vitamin, mineral or herb. For example, compounds like phosphatidylserine, glucosamine and several abbreviated substances like DHEA and SAMe belong to this new heading of natural medicines. These compounds cannot be classified into a single category, are relatively new to the market, and are still in the testing process. While their origins may be from natural sources, it's important to understand that many of them are reproduced in laboratories.

The current thrust toward natural healing or the pursuit of wellness through supplementation reflects our penchant for becoming proactive when it comes to personal health issues. The tried-and-true principles of natural healing are nothing new. For centuries they have been based on the following ideals:

- using the healing power of nature
- doing no harm to the patient
- identifying and treating the cause of disease, not just symptoms
- promoting the role of health practitioner as teacher and healer

Keep in mind, that the use of any natural therapy takes time and patience. Overnight results are not the rule. The secret to tapping into natural healing hinges on our willingness to learn what compounds are effective and how to use them properly. I sincerely hope this pocket guide will enable you to make wise choices concerning the use of natural therapies to fight disease, maintain health and promote longevity.

The Dietary Supplement Renaissance

In 1996 alone, Americans spent more than $6 billion on dietary supplements; and at the turn of the century, sales topped $20 billion. In fact, more than half of all Americans take some kind of nutritional supplement. Having said that, our vigorous pursuit of wellness demands that we learn how to separate fact from fiction, not only to protect our health, but our pocketbooks as well.

Products marketed as "dietary supplements" include a diverse range of compounds, from traditional nutrients, such as vitamins or minerals, to high-potency free amino acids, botanicals, enzymes, animal extracts, and bioflavonoids, some of which have no scientifically recognized role in nutrition.

The remarkable trend toward alternative medicine has prompted a dramatic shift to the merger of traditional and complementary medicine; hence a new term has emerged—integrative medicine (using the best of both to promote health and fight disease). This approach offers a much more comprehensive option for the treatment of disorders.

Using appropriate supplements has a great deal to offer, especially for conditions that mainstream medicine has failed to cure or manage. Overusing or misusing supplements, however, can do more damage than good. That's where supplement savvy comes in.

Today's Science Validates Yesterday's Medicines

While our primitive forefathers lacked modern-day validation for their medicinal practices, today we know that their choices were based in solid science. For example, ancient Greek and Roman physicians used liver extracts to treat poor eyesight. Today we know that liver is rich in vitamin A, which prevents the development of night blindness. The same type of correlation applies to vitamin C depletion and scurvy, low iron levels and anemia, thiamine deficiency and diseases like beri beri.

During the 1940s, vitamin D was added to milk to help prevent childhood rickets, a devastating disease that deformed the bones of countless children. While the disease has virtually disappeared, a vitamin D deficiency still plagues many middle-aged and older adults, contributing to the loss of bone (osteoporosis). Likewise, iodine has been routinely added to salt since 1930 to prevent goiter (an enlargement of the thyroid gland). The widespread availability of iodized salt has all but eliminated the disorder. For over fifty years, white flour, cornmeal, and white rice have been enriched with three B-vitamins; thiamin, riboflavin, and niacin, along with iron. In 1998, folic acid was also added.

While taking nutritional supplements may still raise a few eyebrows among physicians, the practice is well supported by scientific data. For example, a recent study conducted by scientists at the Harvard School of Public Health reported that taking 100 IU of vitamin E can reduce the development of heart disease by up to 40 percent. I don't know about you, but I don't typically eat the twenty cups of spinach or ten pounds of asparagus required to supply this much vitamin E.

In addition, the more we learn about diet and health, the more confused we can become. For example in the1970s, physicians discovered that Eskimos living in the Arctic had low levels of cardiovascular disease in spite of their consumption of fatty, high-cholesterol fish.

In time, the correlation between fish consumption and low rates of heart disease was seen elsewhere. Upon closer investigation, scientists concluded that the heart-protective omega-3 polyunsaturated fatty acids found in fish oil accounted for the seemingly contradictory data.

More recently, groups of highly respected scientists have concluded that the hypericum content of St. John's wort does indeed elevate mood and that compounds found in herbs like echinacea and goldenseal fight infectious organisms. Saw palmetto is openly prescribed by doctors for prostate disease, and ginkgo biloba and vinpocetine have proven memory enhancing effects. Data continues to accrue on countless other herbs and compounds supporting their therapeutic use. Little known immune boosters like Transfer Factor are gaining impressive credentials, and everyday new compounds emerge.

Why I Believe In Supplementation

Today, scientific evidence supporting dietary supplementation is overwhelming. For example, studies say using a vitamin and mineral supplement during pregnancy could cut in half two of the primary causes of infant death: severe birth defects and low birth weight. Did you know that zinc is involved in at least eighty to ninety metabo-enzymatic reactions; many of which determine immune function. Obviously a zinc deficiency means that the immune system will be compromised.

Eating on the run, choosing sweet, fatty foods as meal replacements and using caffeine for energy are more the rule than the exception. Unquestionably, most Americans are not getting the recommended daily allowances (RDA) of important nutrients. Moreover, RDA standards are not always adequate. Even though the standard is now called RDI (Reference Daily Intake), it still fails to address worst-case health scenarios. Using a good multivitamin supplement only makes good sense. In addition, learning to add other single micronutrients according to your individual needs and your gender is probably wise. While we can work on improving our eating habits, data shows that even in a best-case scenario they probably won't be good enough.

Women are especially prone to nutrient deficiencies because they often restrict calories, lose iron through their periods, and frequently take birth control pills, which can lower certain nutrient levels. RDA standards often aren't adequate for those battling high stress or chronic disease.

At this writing, emerging statistics show that significant deficiencies in the B-vitamins, chromium, iron, selenium, calcium, etc. exist in this country. In the area of cancer alone, deficiencies in vitamin A, C, and E have all been linked to increased risk. Copper and zinc depletions profoundly impact immunity, and low chromium levels are thought to be responsible for cholesterol escalation and many blood sugar disorders. A lack of selenium can predispose us to heart disease, and low magnesium can significantly contribute to PMS.

Data strongly suggests that using nutritional supplements now could save millions of dollars in health care services later. For example, making sure that we get adequate and absorbable amounts of calcium/magnesium in our younger years could help prevent the high incidence of hip fractures we see in our older populations; a fact that ends up costing the system millions of dollars in medical care costs.

Recent studies have found that in some diseases like breast cancer the aggressive use of nutritional antioxidants, essential fatty acids and coenzyme Q10 has resulted in significant remission. Concerning the use of supplements for disease like cancer, B. Levin, in the winter 1995 *Quarterly Review of Natural Medicine* stated, "This study should help convince us that serious health compromise can increase the need for certain nutrients. This study also suggests a primary role for aggressive nutritional supplementation in the treatment of breast cancer." Simply stated, taking supplements is wise.

A Few Rather Surprising Facts

The *Journal of Clinical Nutrition* reported that less than 10 percent of those surveyed eat a balanced diet, and up to 80 percent of exercising women and many children have iron-poor blood. Consider the following revelations that only further support our need for supplementation:

- Many diets in the U.S. provide only half the recommended amounts of folic acid.
- Only one person in five consumes adequate levels of vitamin B6.
- Nine out of ten diets are marginal in chromium as well as vitamin A, C, B1, B2, B6, iron, copper, and zinc.
- As many as 20 percent of people hospitalized for depression are lacking vitamin B-6.
- One ambitious one-day survey of 12,000 people showed that 41 percent ate no fruit, and only 25 percent reported eating a fruit of vegetable that contained vitamin C or A.
- A U.S. study showed that adolescents consumed diets that were low in several essential vitamins and minerals related to increased incidence of chronic diseases like ADD, chronic fatigue, depression and suicide.

- 72 percent of adult Americans fall short of the recommended dietary allowance for magnesium.
- The average calcium consumption in the U.S. and Canada is two-thirds the RDA of 800 mg.
- 59 percent of our calories are coming from potentially nutrient-poor food sources (e.g., soft drinks, white bread, snack foods). These poor food choices result in a sub-optimal status for essential vitamins and minerals.
- A recent study says that most of our children rely on cold sugar cereal as their primary source of vitamins and minerals.

Even if we tried to meet the RDA, now referred to as the Reference Daily Intake standards, with food alone, our diets would typically have to consist of several portions of whole grain products, several servings of fresh, raw fruits and vegetables, legumes, nuts, or other protein sources and adequate, absorbable sources of calcium. Very few of us eat like this every day.

Daily Values: A New Term

Daily value is a new term found on food an supplement labels. It refers to the amount of a nutrient that is provided by a single serving of a food item. New daily values are based on two sets of standards: the Reference Daily Intake standards, which suggest the recommended level of intake for most vitamins and minerals, and the Daily Reference Values, which are used for other nutrients that impact health.

The following are the daily values based on Daily Reference Values:

Nutrient Daily Value

Nutrient	Daily Value
Total Fat	65 grams (based on 30% of 2,000 calories)
Saturated Fat	20 grams (based on 8%–10% of 2,000 calories)
Cholesterol	300 milligrams
Total Carbohydrate	300 grams (about 60% of 2,000 calories)
Fiber	25 grams
Sodium	2,400 milligrams
Potassium	3,500 milligrams
Protein	50 grams (about 10% of 2,000 calories)

*DRV for protein does not apply to certain populations; Reference Daily Intake (RDI) for protein has been established for these groups: children 1 to 4 years: 16 g; infants under 1 year: 14 g; pregnant women: 60 g; nursing mothers: 65 g.

The following are the daily values based on Reference Daily Intake:

Nutrient Daily Value

Nutrient	Daily Value
Vitamin A	5,000 IU
Vitamin C	60 milligrams
Vitamin D	400 IU
Vitamin E	30 IU
Thiamin	1.5 milligrams
Riboflavin	1.7 milligrams
Niacin	20 milligrams
Vitamin B6	2 milligrams
Vitamin B12	6 micrograms
Folic Acid	0.4 milligrams
Biotin	0.3 milligrams
Pantothenic Acid	10 milligrams
Calcium	1,000 milligrams
Iron	18 milligrams
Phosphorus	1,000 milligrams
Iodine	150 micrograms
Magnesium	400 milligrams
Zinc	15 milligrams
Copper	2 milligrams

(IU = international units)

Dietary Supplementation Nixes Nutrient Killers

Even if we all ate wonderfully balanced diets from nutrient-laden food on a regular basis, we need to consider the effects of the following nutrient destroyers:

Stress

Continual stress causes the release of free radicals, which assault our cellular systems, and cortisol, which weakens our immunity. Studies done with people under high stress (caring for Alzheimer's patients in a nursing home) found that their wounds healed much more slowly than a control group. New statistics suggest that as much as 90 percent of all physical illness is stress-related.

Sugar

The average American eats over 125 pounds of white sugar every year. It has been estimated that sugar makes up 25 percent of our daily caloric consumption, with soda pop supplying the majority of that intake. Significant amounts of B-vitamins are actually required to metabolize and detoxify sugar in our bodies. Moreover, when you overload your body with sugar, you can inhibit the assimilation of nutrients from other foods.

Food Storage

Unlike our grandparents, we no longer eat foods in season. Fruits and vegetables are shipped trans-continentally and are often packed in dry ice or in cold storage for extended periods of time. In the process, nutrients are lost.

Synthetic Edibles

New foods and synthetic food substitutes like aspartame and newly emerging "fake fats" like olestra are rapidly dominating our selection of grocery store foods. Fat substitutes can deplete your body of nutrients and significantly interfere with the absorption of fat soluble vitamins like E, A, K and D.

"Anti-foods"

Some of our foods are actually "anti-foods" in that they serve to inhibit or destroy nutrients. Phosphorus found in soft drinks causes the body to lose calcium, and sugar and caffeine deplete the body of B-vitamins and other essential nutrients.

Heavy Physical Demands

Some experts say we expect too much from ourselves. Women are notorious for crowding their day with too much to do, including housework, working outside the home, exercising, dieting, community and church work, etc. Some experts believe that the energy levels we are seeking are totally unrealistic. Ideally, because we demand so much from ourselves, we need to keep our cells well nourished. Realistically, we often fall short of this goal.

Using Caffeine, Alcohol, Nicotine or Drugs

Caffeine stimulates the release of norepinephrine, which can create a temporary energy surge. What is not commonly known is that it also inhibits the body's ability to absorb B-vitamins. In addition, it causes the body to lose magnesium, agitates the nervous system, stresses the adrenal glands and is considered addictive. Birth control pills can also affect B-vitamin levels. Several studies have found that some women who take birth control pills and become depressed have low levels of B-6. If you continually use diuretics, you can develop a sodium or potassium deficiency, and virtually every drug inhibits the action of various nutrients. Naturally, if you smoke or use alcohol, you are destroying nutrients on an even greater scale.

Medical Professionals and Nutritional Supplements

Many health professionals take supplements themselves but do not recommend them to their patients. Interestingly, their better-informed patients take the supplements anyway. Patients who don't take dietary supplements are typically the ones who are the most malnourished.

Viva Vitamins!

Ideally, our diets should provide us with adequate supplies of vitamins. Realistically, this is far from the case. RDA or RDI requirements may be enough to ward off deficiency symptoms, but they rarely address increased nutrient requirements brought on by disease, stress, and environmental toxins. For this reason, vitamin supplementation is recommended, especially in people who suffer from compromised health or require extra endurance.

What Is a Vitamin?

The technical definition of a vitamin is an organic compound that is continually needed by the body in tiny amounts to drive a variety of essential functions. In other words, vitamins supply us with the building blocks of life. They are remarkable micro-compounds designed to initiate and assist in countless biochemical processes that sustain life. Vitamins are intimately linked to enzymes that activate thousands of chemical chain reactions required by each body system to operate. For this reason, vitamins are also called co-enzymes.

Ideally, Mother Nature intended that we get all the vitamins we need from plant or animals sources. Plants utilize a combination of sunlight, air, water and soil-containing minerals to produce a variety of vitamins. Keep in mind that vitamins can be found in organic compounds or produced in the laboratory as imitation compounds. All vitamins sold in this country must meet certain quality standards set by the U.S. Pharmacopeia (USP). Vitamins that are manufactured in other countries still have to meet USP standards to be marketed in the U.S.

Mineral Makings

By contrast, minerals are inorganic compounds that can come from living sources. Unlike vitamins, minerals are obtained from natural sources in their raw state after which they undergo purification in a laboratory setting. Plants absorb minerals from the soil they grow in. It's important to realize that all the vitamins in the world won't do you a bit of good without the catalyzing effect of minerals. Surprisingly, in the midst of unprecedented prosperity, many of our citizens are mineral deficient. Iron deficiencies, for example, are common among American children, and selenium and calcium deficiencies are often seen in older individuals.

Supplemental minerals are commonly combined with other substances (such as amino acids) in order to neutralize their toxicity and make them more absorbable. Supplemental minerals are also subject to the USP standards.

Natural Versus Synthetic

Trying to determine what is the best type of vitamin or mineral can be challenging. When purchasing vitamin and mineral supplements, it's easy to get confused amidst claims that natural is superior to synthetic. For example, natural vitamin E, which is derived from the soybean, is thought to be more effectively retained in body tissues than synthetic varieties. By contrast, while natural sources of vitamin C such as acerola berries are good, synthetic ascorbic acid supplements can be just as effective. Keep in mind that even if a supplement is labeled "natural" it probably went through several processing steps in a laboratory. In some cases, a synthetic vitamin may outshine its natural counterpart. Some studies suggest that the manufactured or synthetic form of folic acid may be better absorbed and assimilated than the folic acid found in green leafy vegetables.

While vitamins can be artificially manufactured, minerals cannot be synthesized. These elements, which are commonly found in the soil and other sources, undergo purification processes for isolation. Mineral sources can vary. For example, calcium can be isolated from oyster shells, eggshells, limestone, calcium-containing coral, etc. You should be aware that minerals are commonly paired with other compounds to lessen their toxicity and make them more absorbable. All vitamins, whether they are synthetic or natural, are manufactured in large plants. Interestingly, six large companies provide the main source of all vitamins, which are subsequently purchased from scores of other supplement companies and used in various potencies and combinations for individual products.

While the debate continues over synthetic versus natural vitamins, it is important to keep in mind that vitamins derived from inorganic chemicals may be combined with undesirable substances like sugar, artificial colors, preservatives, and coal tars. Protein-bound vitamins have been shown to have some advantages, much the same way "chelated" minerals do. Always read label breakdowns and purchase vitamins in dark, protective containers. Use reliable sources for vitamins that are pure and potent, and remember that more is not always better.

Potency of Multiple Vitamin Supplements

Combining a variety of vitamins and minerals to create the optimum mix has made multiple vitamin and mineral supplements very popular. Most of these products offer the minimum of the U.S. Recommended Dietary Allowance (USRDA) for their vitamin selections. Mineral potencies are usually provided at lower than RDA levels. Most multiple products will include a standard array of nutrients including: vitamins A, B-complex, C, D, E, and K, and calcium, magnesium, zinc, iodine and selenium. Iron is optional. You'll notice that phosphorus and sodium are never included because we get more than we can use from our high salt and soda pop laden diets. Some trace minerals such as biotin have no RDA standard but are still considered critical nutrients that contribute to optimal health and disease prevention.

Ideally the micronutrients that should be included in a complete multiple supplement are vitamins A, B-complex (thiamine, riboflavin, niacin and/or niacinamide), folate, pantothenic acid, and biotin, vitamins C, D, E, K and calcium, magnesium, zinc, iodine, selenium, copper, manganese, chromium, molybdenum and possibly iron.

One-a-Day Varieties

What about "one-a-day" multiple products? Usually these supplements are comprised mostly of B-complex vitamins in combination with some vitamin A and vitamin D. They commonly lack other nutrients such as selenium, and vitamin E. Because the whole notion of a one-a-day supplement is to fulfill our nutrient needs, you can get a false sense of security in assuming that one pill has it all. Many of these multiples lack in vitamin C or in calcium or magnesium; hence other pills need to be added to make the formula complete. For this reason, one-a-day packets, which include a more comprehensive assortment of nutrients in stronger potencies may be a better way to go.

Separate Supplements Commonly Added to Multiple Formulas

While multiples are convenient, taking nutrients in separate dosages makes it easier to change the dose of one and not the other. It may also be less expensive, however, you can expect to take from 5 to 12 pills twice daily. Learn to look at potency labels of products and make comparisons, so you get the most for you money. Ask your health practitioner for advice in designing your own individual supplement program.

Nutrient Values Depend on Individual Need

While RDA or RDI guidelines give us somewhere to start, remember that your individual supplement need will vary, depending on your situation. For example, pregnant women need twice as much iron, vitamin D and folic acid than non-pregnant women. If you're nursing, you need more of everything, especially calcium. In fact, you may need more nutrients to stay healthy than you did when pregnant. Likewise, you may need extra vitamin C if you catch everything that comes along, smoke or are over 60. As we grow older, supplementation becomes more crucial because our eating habits usually deteriorate. Many seniors lack calcium, the B-vitamins, selenium and vitamin D. Simply stated, your age, sex and lifestyle impact your daily requirements for vitamins and minerals. Consuming alcohol, engaging in vigorous athletic activity and recovering from surgery or injury can up your nutrient needs. Strict vegetarians are prone to vitamin B-12 deficiencies, and women with heavy periods may need more iron.

Today, the new emphasis is not on supplying our bodies with the minimum amount of nutrients needed to keep us from becoming deficient. Instead, health researchers are looking at levels of nutrients that provide optimal health and disease protection. The use of certain vitamins and minerals to prevent or treat heart disease, cancer and even diabetes is currently under investigation.

A Pill by Any Other Name

Vitamins are available in capsules, tablets or liquids—which, if any, is best? Most people find that capsules are easier to swallow than tablets. Tablets are usually larger and more compressed, and if made properly should dissolve in the stomach. Be aware, however, that some tightly compressed tablets have been known to pass through the intestinal tract intact. Because gel caps dissolve more rapidly, you make experience some nausea if you take your supplement on an empty stomach. Keep in mind also that most capsule coverings are made from animal gelatin. If you are a strict vegetarian, read labels carefully.

Time-Release Supplements

Some supplement products are available in a time-released form. The thinking behind this type suggests that a slow release of vitamins and minerals over a period of time is preferable to an all-at-once approach.

While some studies have shown that time-release vitamin C appears to have a better absorption rate, tests on other vitamins are not yet available. Most time-release products are more expensive. In addition, there is some speculation that the slow release of all nutrients may actually be less effective than a one time boost. Concern over time-release pills dissolving at the right time is also an issue. In the case of vitamin B-3 or niacin, time-release varieties can actually prevent the temporary flushing of the skin, but may tax the liver in some individuals.

When Should You Take Your Supplements?

For the most part, vitamin and mineral supplements should be taken with food, thereby replicating the synergistic action of the wide nutrient profile naturally found in foods. Amino acid supplements are the exception to this rule. In addition, taking vitamins and minerals on an empty stomach may cause nausea. Vitamin C can be taken at any time and unless used in mega-doses (over 5,000 mg), does not cause stomach upset. Powdered varieties of C (ascorbic acid) can be easily added to juice if you need to take higher-than-normal doses. Sometimes, an antagonism or competition for absorption between different nutrients can occur. For example, copper and zinc, and iron and vitamin E compete. This phenomena is usually not a serious concern when taking large doses of supplements.

Tips to Make the Taking Easier

Interestingly, if you have trouble swallowing pills, taking them with a thick drink such as apricot or tomato juice can help. Waiting until you are really thirsty also makes it easier to swallow supplements. I like to place all my daily pills in a compartmentalized container, one space for each day. This way, I can check the box for that day and make sure that by evening, it is empty. Ice trays, fishing tackle or sewing boxes, and large medicine dispensers work well. Without this kind of system, you would have to open countless bottles daily, which may be a deterrence.

Storing Supplements

Keep all supplements in a cool, dry place. If you leave any supplement in a hot car or suitcase over a period of time, you risk compromising or even destroying its potency. Most products don't need to be refrigerated (exceptions: liquid acidophilus and fatty acids). Keep supplements out of humid places like the bathroom and avoid storing them over the stove, or in a place exposed to sunlight. If you want to extend the life of a supplement, it can be refrigerated or frozen; however, after opening the bottle, cap it quickly to avoid condensation.

Shelf Life

Most supplements have expiration dates. If you use them after this time, they may not be effective. Each nutrient has a different shelf life, and many will still be viable after expiration dates if stored properly. There is no way of knowing. Minerals are quite stable and do not degrade even when stored for long periods of time. Discard any supplement that has become discolored, spotted or smells funny. You can buy a 3 to 5 month supply of supplements if you store them in a cool, dry and dark environment. Always check the expiration date on a supplement bottle before you buy it. If you see a code such as 0201005, it simply means that the expiration date is February 1, 2005.

Chatting about Children's Chewables

Unfortunately, masking the strong taste of B-vitamins for children's chewables means using a sweetener. Sucrose (table sugar) or fructose (fruit sugar) are commonly used and sometimes artificial sweeteners like aspartame (NutraSweet) or saccharin are added. Personally, I prefer natural sugars to synthetic imitations, especially for children. Children's chewables come in all kinds of shapes and colors and can provide good nutritional support for your finicky youngster. One to two daily is usually recommended. Purchase multiples without iron, unless specified by your health care practitioner. Overdosing on iron can pose serious health risks for young children. If you can't get your child to chew these vitamins, liquid varieties can be hidden in juice, milk, etc. Compare the nutrient arrays of different products. A little research goes a long way toward finding the best supplement for your child.

The Herbal Renaissance

Herbal medicine is nothing new. Virtually every culture on earth used plants in medicinal applications. Discorides listed some 700 healing plants in a comprehensive record called *De Materia Medica*. The native people of every continent utilized their local plants for every disease or injury they encountered. In this country, as white settlers pushed the frontier farther west, they learned of Native American plants and how to use them to treat infections and other illnesses. Native Americans gave us herbs like sarsaparilla, black cohosh, sassafras, capsicum, goldenseal, and even echinacea. At the turn of the twentieth century, herbs were still listed in the *Physician's Desk Reference*.

Unfortunately, herbal remedies fell out of favor with the advent of drug manufacturing. The new consensus was that synthetic drug compounds are more effective than plant-based therapies. Today, our dependency on prescription drugs and their potential drawbacks has catapulted us into a great herbal renaissance.

While herbal compounds may have unfamiliar or unscientific-sounding names, be assured that scores of clinical studies support their effectiveness. Moreover, herbal remedies are backed by thousands of years of use. Today, most medicinal herbs come from lush tropical rain forests or specially cultivated herb farms. Herbal compounds may be extracted from the root, bulb, bark, leaf or flower of a plant.

Herbs listed in this guide have been selected for their efficacy and their reputation. Herbs and botanical compounds are technically considered dietary supplements and include processed or unprocessed plant parts. Extracts and essential oils are also derived from plant parts and come in water infusions (teas), tablets, powders, capsules and elixirs. These phyto (plant) medicines are available as single supplements or in combination formulas, which may include other herbs, vitamins, minerals, amino acids, etc.

Today, the search for curative plants continues. Ethnobotanists all over the world continue to study plants in remote areas, hoping to find the cure for cancer and other devastating diseases. Keep in mind that many pharmaceutical drugs have used natural plant compounds as the basis of their chemical design. In the early 1800s, scientists began to isolate healing compounds from plants. For example, from willow bark came aspirin; from poppies, morphine; from cinchona, quinine (used to prevent and control malaria); and from foxglove, digitalis, a commonly used heart medicine. In Germany alone, people have access to over 700 plant-based medicines, and their expense is often covered by health insurance plans. It is estimated that over 70 percent of German physicians routinely prescribe herbal medicines for their patients.

The price the body pays for quicker, more powerful results is risk. It is important to remember that, just like anything in nature, herbs work more slowly than drugs. At the same time, herbs have the ability to target and treat the root causes of disease rather than just mask symptoms. In addition, the positive effects of herbs are usually longer lasting than drug therapies.

The Adaptogenic Action of Herbs

Simply stated, herbs are adaptable, drugs are not. One of the most remarkable qualities of many herbal medicines is that they are adaptogens. An adaptogen can either potentiate or dilute its therapeutic action based on the specific needs of the body. No synthetic drug has that kind of smarts. In addition, while getting to the root cause of many ailments, phytomedicines work to restore the body's overall balance, an ability that eludes even the most sophisticated pharmaceutical drug.

Current Views of Herbal Medicine

Treating disease with herbal remedies is unquestionably proliferating into mainstream medicine. European physicians have prescribed herbs for generations. And here, in this country, new interest in herbs like St. John's wort has prompted physicians to take notice. For this reason, it is vitally important that consumers take advantage of the most current and reliable data concerning botanical medicine. At this writing, herbs are still classified as foods or food additives. Therefore, manufacturing companies cannot legally list any of their therapeutic applications on bottle labels. Exercise caution when selecting herbs and to never assume that because a substance is natural, you can take it in excessive amounts.

Tips for Administering Herbs to Children

Herbs or any other compounds should not be given to children unless supervised by a qualified health practitioner who can recommend the proper dose based on the child's weight. Using herbal extracts or tinctures are the easiest way to give herbs to children. Add extracts and tinctures to juice, water, formula or soft foods such as applesauce and cereal. Because most medicinal herbs are bitter, placing them directly in your child's mouth may cause an unpleasant reaction. You can also place herbal extracts in a teaspoon of jam or other type of syrup to mask the taste. If your child is older and pickier, try making herbal popsicles with herb teas mixed into fruit juice.

Herbs that Should Not Be Given to Children

White willow bark contains salicylate compounds like those found in aspirin and should never be given to a child under twelve during an infection to avoid the risk of Reye's Syndrome. The following herbs have compounds that can be toxic to children, initiate vomiting, prompt unwanted hormonal responses, or are just too stimulating:

aconite, aloe juice, belladonna, blessed thistle, blue cohosh, black cohosh, cayenne pepper, chaparral, comfrey, damiana, dong quai, ephedra, foxglove, green tea, hawthorn, ginseng, licorice, lobelia, mistletoe, nettles, peppermint or mint-based herbs, turmeric, white willow bark, wild yam, yohimbe

Note: Goldenseal and echinacea should not be used for longer than one to two weeks; use it only in child-appropriate doses. If given in excess amounts, the volatile oils found in mint-based teas can cause liver damage in small children and infants.

How to Select Quality Herbal Preparations

Herbal manufactures are not held to the same standards as drug companies. For this reason, the potency and quality of an herbal supplement can vary dramatically. Remember also that herbal medicines are not magic bullets. Unfortunately many plant medicines have been associated with fantastic health claims that are simply not true. As mentioned earlier, by law, herb companies are not allowed to make specific health claims about their products. One of the best ways to make wise herbal purchases is to look for standardized products where the inclusion of active ingredient is guaranteed.

The Profound Importance of Guaranteed Potency

It's vital to purchase natural products from distributors who guarantee potency and offer standardized active ingredients. All the scientific data in the world regarding an herbal medicine is useless if the supplement you purchase is lacking enough of its active constituent. Research tells us that the therapeutic action of an herbal supplement is based on how much of a certain ingredient it possess. Be aware that not every herbal product guarantees potency. Consequently, you may end up wasting your money and time. Of equal importance is the fact that if your herbal supplement fails you, you may conclude that all natural therapies are worthless.

Only purchase herbal supplements that have been standardized and subject to rigorous quality control. Diluted, inert or inactive forms of herbs will not initiate desired physiological reactions. Learning how to recognize good herbal blends is also helpful. The good design of an herbal formula reflects the reputability and expertise of its manufacturer.

Herbal Buying Tips

- Purchase herbs that are pure and have the desired potency. Get them from reliable sources. Large manufacturing companies usually have time-honored reputations and good research and development departments accessible by phone or website.
- Check the botanical name by looking for the genus and species names on the product label. For example there are several kinds of ginseng, each with different medicinal properties.
- Until you are more familiar with combinations, you may want to stick with single herbs. In this way, you can tell exactly how much of the herb you are taking.
- Choose the herbal form that is most effective for what you need. Herbs come in extracts, teas, tinctures, dry capsulized powders, as well as ointments and creams.
- Take recommended dosages, and do not assume that more is always better.
- If you are prone to allergies, are pregnant or nursing, or are taking other drugs for any condition, check with your doctor before using herbs.
- Check expiration dates and keep herbs in a cool, dry place. Tinted containers help to prevent deterioration from light exposure.
- Give children only a fraction of the adult dose depending on their age. Don't give children under the age of two any supplement unless you check with your physician.
- Read the contraindications of certain herbs, and make sure you do not have a condition or are taking drugs that may cause a negative interaction.
- Keep all herbs out of the reach of children.

Remember that herbal medicines are designed to work with the body and usually require consistent use over a long period of time to achieve the desired results.

Note: Wild-crafted herbs are gathered in the wild as opposed to cultivated herbs, which usually have more consistency. Whichever you choose, try to buy herbs from companies that are ecologically minded. Call toll-free numbers and and find out whether herbs are sourced from endangered rain-forest species; and if so, ask whether they are replaced or not. Cultivation farms can help minimize plant and tree stripping.

Safety of Herbal Preparations

When a drug or other substance is considered government approved, it is usually classified as "generally recognized as safe" (GRAS). Just because a medicine is natural, doesn't mean that it should not be taken judiciously. Many herbs in large doses can cause serious side effects and some should not be mixed with other medications. Likewise, people with specific health conditions should not use certain herbs.

Herbal Vocabulary

Therapeutic Actions of Herbs

Adaptogen: Boosts resistance to stress

Alkaloid: A biochemically active therapeutic plant compound that contains nitrogen

Alterative: Cleanses or initiates the removal of waste

Analgesic: Acts as a pain reliever

Anaphrodisiac: Suppresses sexual desire

Androgenic: Stimulates male characteristics by mimicking the effects of testosterone

Anodyne: Reduces the intensity of pain

Antagonist: Opposes the biochemical action of other medicinal agents

Anthelmintic: Kills worms/ parasites

Antacid: Neutralizes acid

Antibacterial: Kills or inhibits the growth of infectious bacteria

Antibilious: Treats jaundice or reduces biliary conditions

Antibiotic: Destroys or controls the growth of infectious organisms

Anticatarrhal: Inhibits formation of mucus

Antiemetic: Treats nausea and vomiting

Antifungal: Destroys or prevents the growth of fungi

Antigalactagogue: Prevents or inhibits the secretion of milk

Antihemorrhagic: Stops or controls bleeding

Anti-inflammatory: Counteracts the inflammatory response

Antilithic: Prevents or helps relieve stones (gallstones, kidney, etc.)

Antineoplastic: Prevents the development, growth or proliferation of malignant cells

Antioxidant: Protects the cells from free radical or oxidative damage

Antipyretic: Reduces fever

Antiseptic: Neutralizes or controls pathogenic bacteria, thereby preventing spread of infection

Antispasmodic: Relieves spasms

Antithrombotic: Prevents or inhibits the formation of blood clots

Antitussive: Inhibits coughing

Aperitive: Stimulates the appetite

Aphrodisiac: Enhances sexual desire

Aromatic: Contains essential volatile oils, which exert a number of therapeutic actions

Astringent: Constricts blood vessels or exerts a binding effect

Bitter: Stimulates digestive secretions and appetite

Calmative: Calms central nervous system

Carminative: Relieves intestinal gas and promotes peristalsis

Cataplasm: Another term referring to a poultice

Cathartic: Acts as strong laxatives

Cholagogue: Stimulates bile flow from the gallbladder into the duodenum

Demulcent: Soothes and heals inflamed mucous membranes

Depurative: Purifies the blood by boosting the removal of waste

Diaphoretic: Promotes perspiration

Diuretic: Increases the formation and flow of urine

Emetic: Initiates vomiting

Emmenagogue: Stimulates or regulates menstrual flow and should also be avoided in pregnancy

Expectorant: Promotes the liquification and removal of phlegm from the respiratory tract

Febrifuge: Reduces fever

Galactogogue: Stimulates the production and flow of milk

Hepatic: Supports and stimulates liver and gall bladder function and promotes bile secretion

Hydragogue: Promotes the watery evacuation of the stool

Immunostimulant: Enhances or boosts the body's defense systems

Lithotriptic: Dissolves urinary stones

Nervine: Supports the nervous system either through stimulation or sedation

Oxytocic: Stimulates uterine contractions

Parturient: Stimulates uterine contractions and may induce labor

Prophylactic: Works to prevent infection and disease

Purgative: Causes evacuation of the stomach and bowel

Rubefacient: Stimulates blood flow to the skin surface, causing redness

Resolvent: Reduces swelling and inflammation

Restorative: Contributes to the restoration of health, strength and homeostasis

Sialagogue: Promotes the secretion of saliva

Soporific: Induces sleep

Stomachic: Acts as tonics to the stomach

Styptic: Contracts blood vessels and stops bleeding

Sudorific: Promotes perspiration

Taeniafuge: Helps to expel worms

Tonic: Restores and nourishes body systems

Vasoconstrictor: Constricts blood vessels

Vermifuge: Promotes the expulsion or destruction of intestinal worms

Vulnerary: Assists in wound healing by stimulating new cell growth

Types of Herbal Preparations

Bath: Herbal therapy through water-based infusions using immersion or osmosis

Bolus: The use of powdered herbs mixed with cocoa butter for suppository application; also called pessaries

Capsules: Dry powdered herbs encased in gelatin capsules

Cerate: A waxy, fatty, herb-containing medium resembling an ointment with a high melting point

Compresses: Decoctions or herbal infusions soaked into a cloth which is externally applied

Creams: Herbal extracts presented in a water or oil base for absorption through the skin

Decoctions: Liquid herbal preparations made by simmering herbs, thus dissolving their medicinal agents

Douches: Herbal decoctions or infusions administered vaginally

Electuaries: Herbal agents mixed in a sweet, edible base such as honey

Elixirs: Herbs carried in a thin, syrupy liquid

Enemas: Herbal decoctions or infusions delivered to the colon through the rectum

Eyewashes: Strained herbal decoctions or infusions used with an eye-cup for eye conditions

Extracts: Herbs added to oil, vinegar or alcohol mediums

Fomentation: Herbal decoctions or infusions applied hot on a cloth for external conditions

Gargle: Herbal decoctions or infusions gargled for sore throat, gingivitis, etc.

Glycerites: Individual herbal constituents placed in sweet, hydrolyzed vegetable fat

Granules: Pellets, usually made of sugar, combined with herbal agents and dissolved in liquid

Infusions: Plant parts steeped in boiling water for external or internal use

Mucilages: Herbs mixed with water to create a slippery substance for external application

Ointments: Petroleum jelly, lard, lanolin, wax, etc used as a medium for herbal application

Pessaries: (See Bolus)

Plasters: Herbs mixed into a sticky base, which is spread on cotton clot for external application

Poultice: Mashed or ground herbs mixed with liquid to make a thick, topical spread

Powders: Herbs dried and ground for encapsulation or extracts

Salves: Also known as balms, herbs mixed with beeswax or oil for topical use

Sinus Snuff: Powdered herb mixture designed for nasal inhalation

Spray: Herbal decoctions or extracts in spray form

Succus: Fresh herb juice often preserved with alcohol

Syrups: Herbs contained in a sweet medium like honey or maple syrup

Tincture: Concentrated herbal extracts usually kept in vinegar or alcohol medium

Vinegars: Herbs dissolved and kept in vinegar

Single Herb Profiles

Alfalfa *(Medicago sativa)*

Overview: An herb rich in minerals and vitamins, especially iron and vitamin K, alfalfa is considered an estrogen precursor. Its name comes from the Arabian *al-fac-facah*, for "father of all foods." It has a high nutritional profile and has historically been used for kidney problems, boils and irregular menstruation.

Therapeutic Applications: allergies, anemia, arthritis, asthma, Bell's palsy, blood disorders, bursitis, high cholesterol, digestive disorders, poor appetite, fatigue, gout, lactation, kidney disorders, morning sickness, menopause, nausea, Cushing's disease, rheumatism, ulcers, urinary tract infections

Scientific Updates: Alfalfa contains eight essential amino acids, is a rich source of vitamin B12 and natural fluoride, contains phytoestrogens and has a high chlorophyll content. It has also demonstrated an antirheumatic effect, lowers cholesterol, and improves overall health and vigor. Recent French studies have found that alfalfa can reduce tissue damage caused by radiation exposure. In addition, it has also known antibacterial and antitumor properties. Because it can neutralize acidity, alfalfa is also beneficial for bladder and urinary tract infections.

Safety: Most powdered alfalfa plant parts contain L-cavanine, a compound that can cause abnormal blood cell counts, recurrence of lupus or spleen problems. Heating alfalfa can eliminate this potential risk. People with lupus should avoid alfalfa in any form. Due to its estrogenic effects, alfalfa is not recommended for pregnant or nursing women or young children. In addition, the high vitamin K content in alfalfa could, in theory, make the drug warfarin (Coumadin) less effective. Alfalfa sprouts can also house bacteria that can cause food poisoning.

Special Instructions: No therapeutic dose of alfalfa has been established. Some health practitioners recommend dosages ranging from 500 to 1,000 mg of the dried leaf daily or 1 to 2 ml of tincture. Bulk alfalfa can be used in tea preparations (1 to 2 teaspoons per cup, steeped in boiling water for fifteen minutes). If possible, look for products that are free of canavanine.

Product Availability: Look for supplements with 2 to 3 percent saponins. Alfalfa sprouts provide a fresh source of the plant. Alfalfa is also available in bulk powders, capsules, liquid extracts and tablets. Powders are often added to green drinks.

Complementary Agents: acerola cherry, uva ursi, juniper, parsley, buchu, cornsilk, marshmallow, cranberry, vitamin C, bioflavonoids, proanthocyanidins, vitamin A, B-complex, calcium/magnesium, marine lipids, acidophilus

References

De Froment, P. 1974. Unsaponifiable substance from alfalfa for pharmaceuticals and cosmetic use. *French Patent* 2:187,328.

Hwang et al. 2001. Soy and alfalfa phytoestrogen extracts become potent low-density lipoprotein antioxidants in the presence of acerola cherry extract. *Journal of Agriculture and Food Chemistry* 49(1):308–14.

Tyihak, E., and B. Szende. 1970. Basic plant proteins with antitumor activity. *Hungarian Patent*. p. 798.

Aloe Vera (Aloe barbadensis)

Overview: Aloe vera is a natural astringent plant whose leaves possess healing and laxative properties. It has been traditionally used to heal injured tissue and to cleanse the bowel, and has documented anti-inflammatory and antiseptic properties.

Therapeutic Applications: burns, wounds, minor skin irritations, acne, AIDS, allergies, bed sores, canker sores, chicken pox lesions, colitis, constipation, diabetes, herpes, insect bites and stings, psoriasis, scar tissue, sores, sunburn, gastric ulcers, leg ulcers, asthma

Scientific Updates: Current research shows that aloe vera expedites the healing of second degree burns by inhibiting inflammation while stimulating tissue healing. Other recent studies have confirmed that aloe has the ability to fight against a variety of bacteria and fungi. Because it has impressive antimicrobial properties, it makes an excellent preparation for the treatment of burns. It has shown antibacterial properties against the staphylococcus and streptococcus types. It has also shown significant antiviral activity against HIV. In addition, aloe vera has shown itself to be an immune system stimulant, an anti-inflammatory agent, a booster of tissue repair and a compound that can actually lower blood sugar.

Safety: Topical application of the gel is considered safe, unless one is allergic to aloe. For serious burns, the gel may actually inhibit proper healing. As a laxative, if aloe is used for more than ten consecutive days, it can cause dependency and may even worsen constipation. Overdoing oral doses of aloe vera may cause cramping and diarrhea.

Special Instructions: For constipation, you can take 50 to 100 mg of aloe vera daily for a maximum of a week. For minor burns, you can apply aloe gel to the affected area three to six times daily. The gel can also be used internally at 30 ml three times daily.

Product Availability: Aloe vera comes in a concentrate form, as a juice, in capsules or as a naturally occurring gel. Look for products that contain 100 percent pure aloe vera and no additives. Having a fresh plant provides a ready source of gel, which is obtained by slitting a leaf lengthwise and applying its contents to the affected area.

Complementary Agents: vitamin E, tea tree oil, St. John's wort (in topical form)

References

Kahlon et al. 1991. Inhibition of AIDS virus replication by acemannan in vitro. *Molecular Biotherapy* 3:127-35.

Lorenzetti, L. 1964. Bacteriostatic property of aloe vera. *Journal of Pharmacological Science* 53:1287.

Robson et al. 1935. Myth, Magic, Witchcraft or Fact: Aloe Vera Revisited. *Journal of Burn Care and Rehabilitation* 3:157-62.

Shelton, R. 1991. Aloe Vera, its chemical and therapeutic properties. *International Journal of Dermatology* 30:679-83.

Somboonwong et al. 2000. Therapeutic effects of Aloe vera on cutaneous microcirculation and wound healing in second degree burn model in rats. *Journal of the Medical Association of Thailand* Apr. 83(4): 417-25.

Artichoke *(Cynara scolymus)*

Overview: As one of the oldest and most respected plants, the artichoke was first grown in Ethiopia. Considered a delicacy for the king's table, its medicinal uses are considerable. Its leaves have been used as a diuretic to stimulate the kidneys and as a "choleretic" to stimulate the flow of bile from the liver and gall bladder. These actions help to explain its use for digestion problems. In this century scientists isolated a compound from the artichoke leaf called cynarin, which has been used to treat elevated cholesterol.

Therapeutic Applications: indigestion, high cholesterol, liver protection, gallbladder ailments

Scientific Updates: Good scientific evidence supports the use of artichoke to lower LDL cholesterol and to bring the entire cholesterol profile into better ratios. Several animal studies suggest that artichoke protects the liver from damage by chemical toxins and participates in the metabolism of fats.

Safety: People with gallbladder disease or gallstones should use artichoke only under medical supervision. It should not be used by pregnant or nursing women, and its safety in young children or in people with liver or kidney disease remains unknown. People with allergies to related plants in the Asteraceae family, such as arnica or chrysanthemums, should not use artichoke or cynarin preparations.

Special Instructions: Germany's Commission E recommends using 6 grams of the dried herb or its equivalent in capsules divided into three daily doses.

Product Availability: Look for products made from 100 percent pure artichoke leaves.

Complementary Agents: peppermint oil, ginger, garlic, milk thistle

References

English et al. 2000. Efficacy of Artichoke dry extract in patients with hyperlipoproteine-mia. *Arzneimittelforschung* 50: 260–265.

Kraft, K. 1997. Artichoke leaf extract—recent findings reflecting effects on lipid metab-olism, liver and gastrointestinal tracts. *Phytomedicine* 4:369–378.

Ashwagandha *(Withania somniferum)*

Overview: Ashwagandha belongs to the pepper family and is native to India and Africa. Its roots have a long history of medicinal use in tra-ditional Indian and Ayurvedic medicine as an overall body tonic. The shoots and seeds of the plant were traditionally used to thicken milk in India and were added to Ayurvedic formulas. Molecules in this plant are like steroids, similar to those found in Panax ginseng. For this reason, ashwagandha has also been referred to as Indian ginseng.

Therapeutic Applications: Alzheimer's disease, immune dysfunction, HIV support, stress, viral infections

Scientific Updates: Ashwagandha is considered an immune tonic. It also has anti-inflammatory properties and may enhance memory. Because it is a true adaptogen, it can be used in cases of chronic debility or when endurance and stamina need to be restored.

Safety: At this writing, no side effects have been reported with the use of ashwagandha. Its safe use during pregnancy and when nursing have not been investigated.

Special Instructions: Doses range from 1 to 2 grams daily of the whole herb which can be taken in capsule or as a tea. For tea, boil the roots for twenty minutes and let stand for ten minutes. Two to three cups daily are recommended. You may also use 2 to 4 milliliters of tincture or fluid extracts of the herb daily.

Product Availability: Because the roots take time to boil into a tea, cap-sulized versions of this herb are more convenient.

Complementary Agents: ginseng, ginkgo, vinpocetine, brewer's yeast, B-complex , protein supplements, green drinks

References

Anabalgan, K. and J. Sadique. 1981. Anti-inflammatory activity of Withania somnifera. *Indian Journal of Experimental Biology* 19: 245–49.

Bhattacharya et al. 1995. Effects of glycowithanolides from Withania somnifera on an animal model of Alzheimer's disease and perturbed central cholinergic markers of cognition in rats. *Phytotherapy Res* 9:110–13.

Bone, K. 1996. *Clinical Applications of Ayurvedic and Chinese Herbs.* Queensland Australia: Phytotherapy Press.

Astragalus, Huang qi *(Astragalus membranaceus)*

Overview: Considered an adaptogenic herb, astragalus has impressive immune boosting properties and fights against both bacterial and viral invaders. In addition, it appears to help increase resistance to disease organisms, especially for cancer patients who have weakened immunity. Some studies suggest it actually shortens the duration of colds and flu. Chinese practitioners have also turned to astragalus for its remarkable healing actions.

Therapeutic Applications: immune dysfunction, HIV, overactive bladder, cancer, chronic diarrhea, diabetes, shortness of breath, herpes, weakness, night sweats, respiratory diseases (colds and flu), boils and sores, fibromyalgia, stress, chronic fatigue syndrome, poor appetite, hypertension, insomnia,

Scientific Updates: Astragalus supplementation in nineteen cancer patients found that the treatment helped restore normal immune function in most test subjects. Data shows that astragalus supplementation actually increased the life span of people with cancer. Extracts of astragalus have also been shown to improve atherosclerosis, hyperthyroidism, diabetes, hepatitis and herpes.

Safety: Astragalus is generally regarded as safe, although its effects during pregnancy and lactation and for those with kidney or severe liver disease have not been established. High doses may cause mild gastrointestinal distress or allergic reactions.

Special Instructions: You can boil up to 30 grams of dried root for twenty minutes to make tea. You may also purchase alcohol and water based standardized astragaloside products, although no percentage as yet been established.

Product Availability: You may use the sliced and whole root (huang qi) to make tea or take the herb in a tincture or capsulized form.

Complementary Agents: echinacea, goldenseal, cordyceps, olive leaf, garlic, ginseng, transfer factor, zinc, vitamin A, vitamin C with bioflavonoids

References

Kamei et al. 2000. The effect of a traditional Chinese prescription for a case of lung carcinoma. *Journal of Alternative and Complementary Medicine* Dec. 6(6): 557–9.

Sun et al. 1983. Immune restoration and/or augmentation of local graft versus host reaction by traditional Chinese medicinal herbs. *Cancer* 52: 70–73.

Bilberry *(Vaccinium myrtillus)*

Overview: Suited for intestinal upsets such as diarrhea and irritated intestinal mucosa, this herb is most famous for its ability to improve eyesight. Bilberry helps to manage eye disorders caused by weak capillaries due to its anthocyanin content. European practitioners use this herb for certain types of blindness, especially when related to diabetes. It also helps prevent bruising and may lower the risk of high-blood-sugar-related complications.

Therapeutic Applications: blood sugar, bruising, diabetes, diarrhea, eyesight, gallstones, hemorrhoids, kidney stones, circulatory insufficiency, hypoglycemia, night blindness, urinary disorders, varicose veins, macular degeneration, maculitis, retinitis pigmentosa, retinopathy, glaucoma and cataracts

Scientific Updates: Bilberry is considered an herbal antioxidant that helps to inhibit free-radical damage in human tissue. Studies have found that bilberry extract can kill or inhibit the growth of certain fungi and bacteria. Bilberry is also effective in cases of diarrhea and intestinal upset and has been found to inhibit the growth of cancer cells in laboratory experiments.

Safety: Diabetics should check with their doctor before taking this herb.

Special Instructions: Doses of bilberry range from 300 to 500 milligrams daily. You may also use a 25 percent extract containing up to 160 milligrams, three times daily. The dried fruit can be taken at 20 to

60 grams daily or 100 to 300 grams of fresh bilberries. Capsulized versions can be used at 80 to 100 milligrams three times daily.

Product Availability: Look for standardized products with guaranteed anthocyanosides standardized from 25 to 36 percent anthocyanosides. Fresh bilberry fruit is difficult to find. The leaves of this plant can be toxic, so use only the fruit portion of this plant.

Complementary Agents: vitamin C with bioflavonoids, grapeseed extract, goldenseal, fenugreek, gimnema, blueberry, proanthocyanidins, vitamin A, beta-carotene, chromium, bee pollen, bee propolis

References

Alternative Medicine Review 2001 Apr. 6(2): 141-66.

Bomser, J. 1996. In vitro anticancer activity of fruit extracts from Vaccinium species. *Planta Medica* Jun. 62(3): 212-6.

Flynn, Rebecca and Mark Roest. *Your Guide to Standardized Herbal Products.* Prescott Arizona: One World Press. p. 4.

Head, K. Natural therapies for ocular disorders, part two: cataracts and glaucoma.

Black Cohosh (*Cimicifuga racemosa*)

Overview: The antispasmodic properties of this herb have made it a favorite botanical remedy for menstrual cramps, muscle spasms, and coughs. It is also believed to stimulate estrogen synthesis, making it a desirable supplement for menopause. In fact, some women have been able to use this herb instead of synthetic estrogen replacement.

Therapeutic Applications: PMS, hormonal imbalances, stress, nervousness, muscle cramping, menopause, lung congestion, inflammatory conditions, hypertension, muscle spasms, rheumatoid arthritis, osteoarthritis, sciatica, neuralgia, leg cramps, endometriosis; menstrual cramps, heavy menstrual bleeding, irregular periods, menopausal symptoms

Scientific Updates: Black cohosh may offer an estrogenic benefit for post-menopausal women. Modern research supports the use of black cohosh for hypertension and cardiovascular disorders. Black cohosh can help to tranquilize an excited nervous system. Recently, the value of black cohosh as a uterine tonic has been supported by clinical research. Current experimentation strongly suggests that black cohosh

also has anti-inflammatory pro...
and smooth muscles and is effec...
Russians have recently approved...
tral nervous system tonic and as a...

Safety: Do not use this herb if p...
should not be taken for longer than...
a doctor's supervision. This herb...
upset, diarrhea, abdominal pain, hea...
and blood pressure. Avoid large doses...
blood sugar. Its safety in young children...
kidney disease is not known.

Special Instructions: The standard dosage of ... ...is one or two
capsules daily of a standardized extract th... ...ntains 1 mg of 27-
deoxyacteine per pill.

Product Availability: Black cohosh is available in tablets, capsules, and
tincture. Don't confuse black cohosh with blue cohosh *(Caulophyllum
thalictroides)*, which has potentially dangerous side effects.

Complementary Agents: squaw vine, soy isoflavones, red clover, calcium, natural progesterone cream, folic acid

References
Duke, James. 1985. *Handbook of Medicinal Herbs.* Boca Raton, FL: CRC Press. p. 120.

Murray, Michael N.D., and Joseph Pizzorno, N.D. 1991. *Encyclopedia of Natural Medicine.* Rocklin, California: Prima Publishing. p. 462.

Pick, M. 2000. Herbal treatments for menopause. Black cohosh, soy and micronized progesterone. *Advanced Nurse Practitioner* May 8(5):29–30.

Black Walnut *(Juglans nigra)*

Overview: Rich in organic tannins, this herb has antifungal and astringent properties which predispose its use for parasitic infections, skin
fungi and other skin eruptions. It has a rich history of traditional use
for stubborn parasitic and fungal infections which are often resistant
to drug therapy. It also has impressive healing properties for bruises,
relieves constipation and is considered a natural antiseptic.

Therapeutic Applications: athlete's foot, boils, ringworm, herpes, yeast

...d sores, eczema, fungus, gum disease, ...worm, tuberculosis, bruises, constipation,

...es: Recent research strongly suggests that black walnut ...gal properties as well as an antiseptic action. Clinical stud-... also found that certain constituents in black walnut have anti-...cer properties. These properties show that viruses and parasites may be linked to malignancies. The high tannin content of the herb is primarily responsible for its ability to expel worms and parasites. Black walnut has also been shown to be a specific for treatment for candida.

Safety: Use in appropriate amounts as directed. Pregnant or nursing mothers should not use this herb. Its safety for children has not been established.

Special Instructions: For liquid extracts taking 1/4 tsp with water three times daily is customary.

Product Availability: Black walnut can be purchased as a tincture, extract or in capsulized form.

Complementary Agents: garlic, cascara sagrada, buckthorn, pumpkin seeds, red clover, culver root, acidophilus, vitamin A, B-complex, pantothenic acid

References

Bhargava et al. Antitumor activity of juglans nigra (black walnut) extractives. *Journal of Pharmaceutical Sciences* 57(10): 1674-1677.

Ody, Penelope. 1993. *The Complete Medicinal Herbal.* New York: Dorling-Kindersley. p. 71.

Ritchason, Jack. 1994. *The Little Herb Encyclopedia.* Pleasant Grove, Utah: Woodland Publishing. p. 30.

Bladder Wrack *(Fucus vesiculosis)*

Overview: As a member of the seaweed family, this herb is found on the coasts that border the Baltic Sea as well as the Atlantic and Pacific oceans. Traditionally used as a food staple in Asian cultures, bladder wrack has traditionally been utilized for its rich iodine content, which greatly contributes to thyroid gland health. It is also rich in alginic acid, which can help buffer excess stomach acid in cases of heartburn. Alginic acid works as a natural laxative as well.

Therapeutic Applications: hypothyroidism, heartburn, constipation, atherosclerosis, immune stimulation, rheumatic joints

Scientific Updates: While there are no specific studies on this particular herb, the nutritive and medicinal value of seaweed plants is well established. Various studies support their ability to stimulate immune response, to lower cholesterol levels and to inhibit the formation of blood clots. Its high iodine content also makes it a tonic for a sluggish thyroid.

Safety: Because seaweed plants can contain residues of heavy metals such as arsenic, they should not be used by pregnant or nursing women, or by children. In addition, the iodine content of various bladder wrack supplements can greatly vary, making it difficult to know how much iodine is being consumed. Use of this herb can also aggravate acne and may inhibit the absorption of iron. It should not be used by people with hyperthyroidism (overactive thyroid).

Special Instructions: You may find that low alcohol extracts are easier to administer. If possible, look for products harvested in areas that are not heavily industrialized to avoid chemical contamination.

Product Availability: You may find bladder wrack added to kelp preparations, although the herb is available in separate form.

Complementary Agents: kelp, blue-green algae, limu moui

References

Lin et al. 1997. B cell stimulating activity of seaweed extracts. *International Journal of Immunopharmacology* 19(3):135–42.

Murata et al. 1999. Hepatic fatty acid oxidation enzyme activities are stimulated in rats fed the brown seaweed. *Journal of Nutrition* 29(1):146-51.

Nishino et al. 1999. Inhibition of the generation of thrombin and factor Xa by a fucoidan from the brown seaweed Ecklonia kurome. *Thromb Res.* 96(1):37-49.

Blessed Thistle *(Cnicus benedictus)*

Overview: Traditionally this herb was made into a tea and used for constipation and digestive problems. There is some evidence that folk practitioners also recommended the tea to increase the production of milk in nursing mothers. It is also known for its ability to stimulate the appetite.

Therapeutic Applications: anorexia, lack of appetite, lactation, circulatory disorders, blood purification, cancer, constipation, digestive problems, fever, gallbladder disease, gas, headaches, heart problems, hormonal imbalances, lactation, liver ailments, lung diseases, painful menstruation

Scientific Updates: Blessed thistle is an excellent supporting herb for plant combinations. It helps stimulate liver function and ease stomach problems, flatulence and tension headaches. It may also help detoxify the body by promoting perspiration and removing excess fluids. Modern studies have found that blessed thistle contains antibacterial and antiyeast properties. It has also demonstrated an ability to strengthen the spleen and liver and to reduce fevers.

Safety: Ingesting excessive amounts of blessed thistle may cause nausea. Contact with the skin should be avoided. If you are allergic to any member of the daisy plant family, avoid this herb.

Special Instructions: Taking 2 ml of a blessed thistle tincture three times daily is customary. You may also add 2 grams of the loose, dried herb to 1 cup of boiling water and steep for fifteen minutes to make a tea.

Product Availability: If possible, find a product that guarantees sesquiterpene, lactone or cnicin content.

Complementary Agents: lemon grass, sage, slippery elm, chamomile, catnip, peppermint, milk thistle, vitamin C, bioflavonoids, calcium/magnesium, digestive enzymes

References

Barney, Paul M.D. 1996. *Clinical Applications of Herbal Medicine.* Pleasant Grove, Utah:Woodland Publishing. p. 66.

Holmes, Peter. 1989. *The Energetics of Western Herbs.* Boulder, CO:Artemis Press. p. 278.

Weiner, Michael and Janet Weiner. 1994. *Herbs That Heal.* Mill Valley, California:Quantum Books. p. 87.

Blue Cohosh *(Caulophyllum thalictroides)*

Overview: Known also as squaw or papoose root, the use of this herb by Native Americans has generated controversy. Used primarily for gynecologic conditions, this herb gained nortoriety for its ability to induce labor and even cause abortions. Its effectiveness and safety have generated significant concern, and its use is not recommended.

Therapeutic Applications: Despite its risks, blue cohosh is widely pre-scribed by some herbalists and midwives today. It also has a track record for menstrual problems. Due to its potential health risks, it should not be used for any condition.

Safety: Blue cohosh is a toxic herb and should be avoided. Do not use it to induce labor. Some of the compounds found in blue cohosh can constrict coronary vessels, which thereby decreases blood flow to the heart. This dangerous effect to the heart was even thought to pass on to an infant whose mother used blue cohosh to induce labor. The com-ponents of this herb have also been linked to birth defects.

References

Irikura, B. and Kennelly, E. 1999. Blue cohosh: A word of caution. *Alternative Therapies in Women's Health* 1:81–83.

Buchu *(Barosma betulina)*

Overview: Native to South Africa, this plant is famous for its glossy green leaves and strong fragrance. Buchu is a natural astringent herb that helps alleviate high acid urine and is beneficial for the prostate gland. It has been traditionally used for chronic kidney and bladder inflammations and is considered an excellent herbal treatment for the prostate.

Therapeutic Applications: bladder infections, diabetes, kidney disease, prostate disorders, water retention

Scientific Updates: The volatile oil content of buchu enables it to stim-ulate urination while also acting as a urinary antiseptic. Buchu elimi-nates mucus and inflammation and has traditionally been used for cys-titis, pyelitis, ureteritis and prostatitis. Diasophenol contained in buchu has antiseptic properties and is considered to be buchu's most important constituent.

Safety: Buchu is considered safe but has not been tested in pregnant or nursing women.

Special Instructions: If you are taking a combination herbal product for kidney or prostate problems, make sure to drink six to eight glasses of pure water daily.

Product Availability: Buchu is often included in herbal combinations designed to support the kidney and bladder. Although it can be purchased as a single herb, it has a synergistic effect when combined with herbs like cranberry, juniper berry and uva ursi.

Complementary Agents: uva ursi, parsley, cornsilk, cranberry, juniper berry, alfalfa, marshmallow, bee pollen, vitamin C, bioflavonoids, proanthocyanidins, vitamin A, zinc, mineral and electrolyte supplements

References

Grieve, M. 1994. *A Modern Herbal.* New York: Dorset. p. 134.

Simpson, D. 1998. Buchu—South Africa's amazing herbal remedy. *Scottish Medical Journal* 43(6):189-91.

Tyler, V. 1976. *Pharmacognosy. 7th ed.* Philadelphia: Lead and Febiger.

Buckthorn *(Rhamnus frangula)*

Overview: Native to Europe and western Asia, this herb is now grown in North America. Used by the Cherokee tribe for skin problems, buckthorn is considered a purgative herb that stimulates bowel evacuation and strengthens the liver and gallbladder.

Therapeutic Applications: bowel cleansing, cancer, constipation, fever, gallbladder disease, gallstones, liver ailments

Scientific Updates: Buckthorn has been shown to be a significant inhibitor of leukemia in mice studies. Buckthorn contains anthraquinone glycosides, which work to promote colon peristalsis. European studies have confirmed buckthorn's ability to release its active principles in the small intestine rather than the stomach. Recent studies also show that anthroquinones work to protect heart muscle.

Safety: Excessive doses may cause intestinal gripping and diarrhea with nausea or dizziness. Children should not take this herb in large amounts because it can cause kidney damage. Pregnant or nursing women should avoid this herb due to its laxative effect.

Special Instructions: Because buckthorn can cause intestinal cramping, it should be taken as part of an overall bowel formula where its amount is moderated. Taking it with a ginger supplement can help to prevent gripping.

Product Availability: Buckthorn is often combined with cascara sagrada and other laxative herbs. Do not take it as a single herb.

Complementary Agents: cascara sagrada, red clover, pumpkin seeds, culver root, slippery elm, dandelion, black walnut, quassia, senna, ginger, acidophilus, vitamin A, vitamin E, B-complex, bioflavonoids, marine lipids

References

Kupchan, S. and A. Karim. 1976. Tumor inhibitors 114: aloe emodin: antileukemic principle isolated from rhamnus fangula l. *Lloydia* 39:223-224.

Yim et al. 1998. Myocardial protective effect of an anthraquinone-containing extract of Polygonum multiflorum ex vivo. *Planta Medica* 64(7):607-11.

Youngken, H. 1943. *Textbook of Pharmacognosy. 5th ed.* Philadelphia: Balkiston.

Burdock *(Arctium lappa)*

Overview: Found in the pesky burrs that often attach to the fur of dogs and cats, burdock has a long history of medicinal applications. In Japan, burdock root is used to strengthen the immune system; and in China, it was prescribed for respiratory infections, joint pain and boils. Burdock also promotes the healing of sores. It was also a constituent in the famous Hoxsey cancer formula.

Therapeutic Applications: abscesses, acne, boils, carbuncles, blood disorders, cancer, canker sores, chicken pox, colds, constipation, eczema, fever, gout, hemorrhoids, herpes, blood sugar disorders, poison ivy, poison oak, psoriasis, tonsillitis, tumors, gallbladder disease, liver disease, weak immune system

Scientific Updates: Studies have supported the ability of burdock to help restore liver and gallbladder function. In addition, clinical testing has also established both its antifungal and antibiotic properties.

Burdock can lower blood sugar, inhibit certain types of tumors and greatly contribute to the healing of specific skin ailments like leprosy and venereal disease sores. It has known anti-ulcer properties.

Safety: In 1978, the *Journal of the American Medical Association* published a report of Burdock poisoning. Subsequently it was revealed that the herbal product in question was actually contaminated with atropine, a poisonous chemical from an unknown source. Safety in young children, pregnant or nursing women, or those with severe liver or kidney disease has not been established. Be aware that burdock can interfere with iron absorption. If you are taking insulin or oral medications to lower blood sugar, burdock may increase its effect.

Special Instructions: A typical dosage of burdock is from 1 to 2 grams of the powdered dry root taken three times daily. A tea made with 1 tsp of the dried herb per cup of boiling water steeped for ten minutes can also be used.

Product Availability: Burdock can be purchased as a fluid extract, tincture, tea or in capsulized form.

Complementary Agents: chaparral, alfalfa, dandelion, echinacea, yellow dock, Oregon grape, cascara sagrada, buckthorn, blue-green algae, kelp, licorice, milk thistle, aloe vera, vitamin A, B-complex, essential fatty acids, zinc, potassium, lecithin

References

Bryson et al. 1978. Burdock root tea poisoning. Case report involving a commercial preparation. *Journal of the American Medical Association* 239:2157.

Mowrey, Daniel Ph.D. 1986. *The Scientific Validation of Herbal Medicine.* Connecticut:Keats Publishing. p. 2.

Os'kina et al. 1999. The mechanisms of the anti-ulcer action of plant drug agents. *Eksp Klin Farmakol* 62(4):37–9.

Butcher's Broom *(Ruscus aculeatus)*

Overview: A spiny evergreen bush with small leaves describes this botanical. Butcher's broom grows in areas of the Mediterranean and Northern Europe. It resembles the asparagus plant and is also considered a member of the lily family. As a natural vasoconstrictor, butcher's broom strengthens weak blood vessels and discourages the formation of blood clots. It also possesses significant anti-inflammatory properties.

Therapeutic Applications: arteriosclerosis, capillary weakness, diabetic retinopathy, hemorrhoids, inflammation, jaundice, phlebitis, varicose veins, blood clot prevention, leg cramps, gout, jaundice chronic venous insufficiency

Scientific Updates: Research has confirmed the ability of butcher's broom to constrict vessels and inhibit inflammation. Both of these properties make the herb ideal for the healing of fragile capillaries or swollen veins. European practitioners routinely use butcher's broom for any disorder affecting the veins, especially hemorrhoids.

Safety: Butcher's broom is generally considered safe, but an allergy can produce stomach upset.

Special Instructions: If using this herb for venous insufficiency a common dosage is 1,000 mg taken three times daily. Look for standardized extracts and take enough daily to get 50 to 100 mg of ruscogenins. If using a suppository or ointment product, use just prior to going to bed.

Product Availability: Butcher's broom is available in rectal ointments and suppositories designed for hemorrhoids. Encapsulated butcher's broom products are often combined with vitamin C or flavonoids and used for venous insufficiency, especially varicose veins.

Complementary Agents: ginkgo, ginger, horse chestnut, bilberry, vitamin C, bioflavonoids, grape seed or pine bark extract

References

Bouskela et al. 1993. Inhibitory effect of the Ruscus extract and of the flavonoid hesperidine methylchalcone on increased microvascular permeability induced by various agents in the hamster cheek pouch. *Journal of Cardiovascular Pharmacology* 22:225-30.

Flynn, Rebecca M.S. and Mark Roest. 1995. *Your Guide to Standardized Herbal Products.* Prescott AZ: One World Press.

Calendula *(Calendulae flos)*

Overview: This lovely member of the marigold family has traditionally been used to heal wounds and treat various skin inflammations. It also has therapeutic properties suited for fever reduction and can help to regulate the menstrual cycle. Herbal practitioners also recommended calendula flowers for toothaches and neuritis. Its rich content of volatile oils is thought to contribute to its therapeutic properties. In Germany, calendula ointments are widely used for skin problems.

Therapeutic Applications: cuts, scrapes, mouth sores, burns, eczema, diaper rash, sunburn, poison ivy, hemorrhoids, varicose veins

Scientific Updates: Laboratory tests suggest that calendula cream boosts wound-healing while exerting an anti-inflammatory effect. New data also suggests that calendula boosts immune response and does indeed inhibit inflamation in skin disorders.

Safety: Calendula is generally regarded as safe. As is the case with all herbal preparations, some allergic reactions have been reported. Studies have found no significant toxic side effects associated with calendula. High doses, however, may have a sedative effect and may reduce blood pressure. Don't use calendula with sedative, antianxiety, or blood pressure medications.

Special Instructions: Calendula cream should be applied two or three times daily to the affected area. For oral use, pour boiling water over 1 to 2 teaspoons of calendula flowers and allow to steep for fifteen minutes. You may rinse your mouth with this decoction several times daily. If you need a topical application, you can soak a cloth diaper in a calendula decoction and apply it as a compress to the skin.

Product Availability: Calendula creams are convenient and easy to use. You may also find calendula in extracts, tinctures or in capsulized forms.

Complementary Agents (to be used topically): St. John's wort, aloe vera, chamomile, chickweed, goldenseal

References

Amirghofran et al. 2000. Evaluation of the immunomodulatory effects of five herbal plants. *Journal of Ethnopharmacology* 72(1-2):167–72.

Azadbakht, M. 2000. Herbal anti-inflammatory agents for skin disease. *Skin Therapy Letter* 5(4):3–5.

Patrick et al. 1996. Induction of vascularisation by an aqueous extract of the flowers of Calendula offcinalis L. the European marigold. *Phytomedicine* 3:11–18.

Capsicum *(Capsicum annum)*

Overview: Capsicum, also known as *cayenne,* is native to tropical areas of the American continent. It has been extensively used as both a spice and medicinal agent. The Aztecs recommended it for toothaches and parasitic skin diseases and European practitioners used it to shrink swollen lymph glands and to stop bleeding. Cayenne also acts as a diaphoretic, which prompts sweating making it ideal for body cleansing and infection fighting. This herb arrests bleeding, stimulates circulation, strengthens the immune system and acts as an overall catalyst for other therapeutic agents. It also comes in ointment and cream form due to the pain killing properties of capsaicin.

Therapeutic Applications: arthritis, asthma, blood clots, bleeding, bronchitis, colds, fatigue, respiratory disorders, fevers, tonsillitis, sore throat, hoarseness, migraines, obesity, circulatory disorders, indigestion, lack of appetite, ulcers, high cholesterol, (joint, nerve [neuralgia[and muscle pain in topical form)

Scientific Updates: Capsicum may actually protect your stomach from possible damage from NSAIDs (nonsteroidal anti-inflammatory drugs). Its stimulatory action boosts circulation and saliva production which inevitably results in better digestion. Capsicum also increases perspiration, and helps remove toxins from the blood. It promotes the coagulation of blood, so it is useful in preventing external and internal hemorrhaging. Clinical studies have also documented its ability to stimulate the heart and to lower blood serum cholesterol. It also slows fat absorption in the small intestines and increases metabolic rate. Capsaicin ointments (capsaicin is the active ingredient in capsicum) are effective against arthritis and nerve pain.

Safety: Capsicum may cause a burning sensation in the gastrointestinal tract or during subsequent bowel elimination. Start with a small dosage, and work up to the recommended dosage. If pregnant or nursing, check with your physician before using. Avoid contact with the eyes or other mucous membranes and use in recommended dosages only. Its use does not seem to adversely affect stomach ulcers. Don't use capsicum if taking the drug theophylline.

Special Instructions: To avoid stomach upset, take capsicum with food.

For sore throats, a capsicum tincture can be added to hot, salted water as a gargle. Capsicum may be taken at a dosage of one to two standard gelatin capsules one to three times daily.

Product Availability: This herb is often found in combinations designed to fight infection and is also believed to work as a catalyst, which enhances the action of other herbs. Cayenne is available in pills, capsules, and tinctures. In addition, capsaicin ointments are used in topical applications for joint and muscle pain seen in arthritis, fibromyalgia, sprains and strains.

Complementary Agents: peppermint, garlic, ginger, gentian, gotu kola, fennel, saw palmetto, catnip, myrrh, vitamin C, vitamin A

References

Barney, Paul M.D. 1995. *Clinical Applications of Herbal Medicine.* Pleasant Grove, Utah: Woodland Publishing. p. 55.

Holmes, Peter. 1989. *The Energetics of Western Herbs.* Boulder: Artemis Press. p. 322.

Yeoh et al. 1995. Chili protects against aspirin-induced gastroduodenal mucosal injury in humans. *Digestion Discovery Science* 40:580–583.

Cascara Sagrada (Rhamnusd purshiana)

Overview: Also known as California buckthorn, Native Americans were responsible for introducing this sacred bark to sixteenth-century Spanish explorers who called it cascara sagrada. One of nature's most gentle and effective laxatives, this herb stimulates a sluggish colon, while exerting a toning effect. It is one of the most preferred herbal remedies for chronic constipation and is also good for the liver and gallbladder.

Therapeutic Applications: general congestion, constipation, colon disorders, gallbladder disease, gallstones, gas, hemorrhoids, jaundice, kidney stone prevention, liver disorders, parasites, worms

Scientific Updates: Research is underway on cascara's health benefits. The aloe-emodin content of cascara sagrada has shown antileukemic properties and new data confirms that it fights certain types of cancer. The anthraquinones in this herb have also exhibited potent antibacterial properties against intestinal bacteria. The rhein content of cascara is used to expel worms. Cascara increases muscular activity in the large intestine. It can prevent the occurrence of calcium based urinary stones. Cascara sagrada may also help overcome laxative dependency often seen in the elderly.

Safety: At recommended dosages, there is no toxicity. Cascara sagrada should not be used by nursing mothers as its laxative effect can transfer to infant. Pregnant women should avoid using cascara unless directed by their doctor to do so. People with ulcers or irritable bowel syndrome should also check with their doctor before using cascara. Large doses can cause diarrhea and stomach upset.

Special Instructions: It's best to take a cascara supplement just prior to bedtime. It usually produces results in 6 to 8 hours after ingestion.

Product Availability: Look for products that have aged cascara sagrada bark or their effect will be minimal. Cascara is found as a single herb, in laxative combinations, and in several prescription and over-the-counter laxative preparations.

Complementary Agents: dandelion, black walnut, quassia, red clover, garlic, buckthorn, pumpkin seed, marshmallow, slippery elm, culver root, acidophilus, vitamin A, B-complex, vitamin E, calcium/magnesium

References

Marchesi et al. 1982. A laxative mixture in the therapy of constipation in aged patients. *Giornale di Clinica Medica* 63: 850–63.

Pecere et al. 2000. Aloe-emodin is a new type of anticancer agent with selective activity against neuroectodermal tumors. 60(11):2800–4.

Ritchason, Jack. 1994. *The Little Herb Encyclopedia.* Pleasant Grove, Utah: Woodland Publishing. p. 30.

Catnip *(Nepeta cataria)*

Overview: Catnip grows in various areas of North America and got its name from its legendary effect of producing a delirious state in felines. It is most famous for its sedative action in humans and is still used as a tea in England. By acting as a natural antispasmodic, catnip helps to alleviate gas pain and is a favorite treatment for infantile colic. It also promotes therapeutic perspiration during fevers and calms the central nervous system.

Therapeutic Applications: colic, coughs, intestinal gas, bloating, diarrhea, stomach cramping, insomnia, colds, flu, fevers, pain

Scientific Updates: Today catnip is sometimes called "Nature's Alka-Seltzer" due to its ability to aid digestion. It also has some antibiotic properties, which may help to control stomach bacteria. Catnip is used for a variety of ailments, including insomnia and anemia. It is rich in organic iron, which helps to build the blood and animal studies have found that it induces sleep.

Safety: Catnip is considered a safe botanical medicine if used appropriately. Because it has mild uterine stimulating actions, it should not be used by pregnant women. Its safety for young children or individuals with severe liver or kidney disease has not been established. It should only be used in very mild occasional doses for infantile colic.

Special Instructions: Catnip tea can be made by adding 1 cup of boiling water to 1 to 2 teaspoons (5 to 10 grams) of the dried herb. Cover and steep the mixture for ten minutes. You may take 2 to 3 cups daily. A teaspoon of the tea can be given to infants with colic in an eyedropper. For coughs, 5 ml of tincture three times per day can be used.

Product Availability: Catnip is available in dried, loose form, as a tincture, extract, or in capsules.

Complementary Agents: ginger, fennel, peppermint, papaya, capsicum, saw palmetto, myrrh gum, calcium carbonate, pepsin, acidophilus

References

Mowrey, Daniel Ph.D. 1986. *The Scientific Validation of Herbal Medicine.* Connecticut: Keats Publishing.

Osterhoudt et al. 1997. Catnip and the alteration of human consciousness. *Vet Hum Toxicol* 39(6):373–5

Cat's Claw *(Uncaria tomentosa)*

Overview: Also known as *uña de gato*, this herb gets its name from the cat-like claws that grow from its large vines. Used in the rainforests of Peru for generations, cat's claw has impressive anti-inflammatory properties. Its alkaloid content makes it ideal for conditions like arthritis and fibromyalgia. It also has the ability to strip the colon walls of accumulated waste and promote intestinal health. Scientists are looking to this herb for its potential in treating cancer and AIDS. It is thought to boost immune response and also has natural antioxidant properties.

Therapeutic Applications: allergies, arthritis, bursitis, cancer, candida, chemotherapy, chronic fatigue syndrome, cirrhosis, Crohn's disease, female hormonal imbalances, fibromyalgia, hemorrhoids, heart disease, inflammation, intestinal disorders, dysfunctional immunity, lupus, parasites, PMS, radiation treatments or exposure, toxic poisoning, ulcers, viral infections, HIV

Scientific Updates: Recent evaluations of this Peruvian rain forest herb have supported its value for treating serious colon disorders. Research also supports the use of cat's claw for immune system stimulation. Two compounds contained in this herb have also demonstrated the ability to inhibit the multiplication of some viruses. Current studies are looking at the herb as a possible treatment for the AIDS virus. Doctors in Peru have successfully used the herb in treating fourteen types of diagnosed cancer. An Italian study in 1992 suggested that it can also stop cells from mutating, which supports its possible use for cancer.

Safety: European studies have shown that cat's claw has extremely low toxicity, even when taken in large doses. It should not be taken, however, by anyone who has undergone a transplant, by hemophiliacs, or by pregnant or nursing women. Taking cat's claw may cause diarrhea or alter bowel consistency in some individuals. Cat's claw may also have contraceptive properties.

Special Instructions: Cat's claw works on the entire system as a tonic and natural detoxifier. The optimum dosage of cat's claw has not been established. Due to the fact that it varies in forms and potency, follow label directions.

Product Availability: Only the inner bark and root of the vine have medicinal value. For this reason, avoid cat's claw products that do not have guaranteed purity. Some products have outer bark, twigs and other plant parts mixed in. These parts do not offer the optimal therapeutic actions. Be aware that due to a surge in sales of this herb, the

Peruvian government has declared it a threatened species and has banned the harvesting of the root. Today, the inner bark is the only part touched and the roots are left. Cat's claw is available as a tincture, in capsules, and as raw bark for tea. Look for products that contain at least a 0.3 percent alkaloid content.

Complementary Agents: pau d'arco, glucosamine, echinacea, cascara sagrada, acidophilus, shark cartilage, slippery elm, blue-green algae, vitamin A, B-complex, vitamin C, bioflavonoids, grape seed or pine bark extract

References

Aquino et al. 1990. Plant Metabolites: structure and in vitro antiviral activity of Quinovic acid glycosides from Uncaria Tomentosa. *Journal of Natural Products* 52(3):559-64.

The Cat's Claw. 1995. *The Energy Times*, May-June, p. 12.

Cerri, R. 1988. New Quinovic Acid Glycosides from Uncaria Tomentosa. *Journal of Natural Medicine* 51(2):257-61.

Steinberg, P. 1994. Uncaria Tomentosa (Cat's Claw): A Wondrous Herb From the Peruvian Rainforest. *Townsend Letter* May 130: 2.

Chamomile *(Matricaria chamomilla, Chamaemelum nobile)*

Overview: This perennial plant has a long history of use as a natural relaxant. Possibly the most popular herbal tea in the world, it was used by ancient Egyptian practitioners to reduce fevers and to treat kidney, liver and bladder diseases. Chamomile also works to soothe the nerves, promote sleep and induce perspiration during fevers. It is also considered a gastrointestinal tonic. In 1921 a topical form of chamomile was introduced in Germany and used to treat a wide variety of skin disorders.

Therapeutic Applications: Internal Uses: insomnia, anxiety, arthritis, menstrual cramps, and gastrointestinal distress Topical Uses: dermatitis, bed sores, poison ivy, eczema, rashes, wound healing, mouth sores

Scientific Updates: Recent studies have confirmed that chamomile works as a uterine tonic, relaxes the nervous system, and interacts positively with other nervine herbs. It has antibacterial properties, can stimulate the liver, and is currently under study for its anticarcinogenic action. Animal research suggests that chamomile extracts can relax the intestines and reduce inflammation. Data also supports its use for skin irritations and rashes.

Safety: Chamomile has no known toxicity, but avoid extreme doses and do not take it for long periods of time. Allergic reactions are rare, but if you are allergic to ragweed, use chamomile with caution. Chamomile also contains naturally occurring coumarin compounds that can act as blood thinners. Don't use this herb if you are taking prescription anticoagulants. Its safety in young children, pregnant or nursing women, or those with liver or kidney disease has not been established.

Complementary Agents: valerian root, skullcap, hops, wood betony, black cohosh, mullein, marshmallow, passionflower, peppermint, vitamin B-complex, vitamin C, vitamin A, calcium/magnesium, melatonin

Special Instructions: Chamomile cream preparations can be applied to affected areas one to five times daily. Chamomile tea is made by pouring boiling water over 2 to 3 heaping teaspoons of flowers and steeping for ten to fifteen minutes in a closed container. Tinctures and pills should be taken according to the directions on the label. Tinctures that have an alcohol base are thought to be the most potent.

Product Availability: Chamomile comes in tinctures, extracts, creams or teas. Because it is a pleasant tasting beverage, the dried, loose form is recommended for making tea.

References

Isaac, O. and G. Kristen. 1980. Old and new methods of chamomile therapy. Chamomile as example for modern research of medicinal plants. *Medizinische Welt* 31:1145–49.

Patzelt-Wenczler et al. 2000. Proof of efficacy of Kamillosan® cream in atopic eczema. *European Journal of Medical Research* 5:171–175.

Yakolev, V. and A. 1969. Von Schlichtegroll. Anti-inflammatory activity of alpha-bisabolol, an essential component of chamomile oil. *Arzneimittel-forschung* 19(4):615–16.

Chasteberry/Vitex *(Vitex agnus-castus)*

Overview: Chasteberry has been used for medicinal purposes since ancient Greece. It's most noted attribute is its ability to stimulate and normalize the pituitary gland, especially its progesterone function. It can produce effects that appear totally contradictory, but it is actually just regulating normal body function. Perhaps its most beneficial use is as a uterine tonic.

Therapeutic Applications: normalizing female hormone levels, dysmenorrhea, premenstrual syndrome, menopausal change regulation, hormone-related constipation, breast pain, infertility

Scientific Updates: Numerous controlled clinical studies have found that vitex is an effective treatment for premenstrual syndrome. Another recent study examined the therapeutic benefits of vitex for women with fertility disorders and recommended it for infertility treatment, noting that thirty-eight out of sixty-seven of the women with fertility disorders achieved pregnancy during the study. Another study found vitex to be a very effective treatment for cyclical breast pain. An extract from the plant has also been found to effectively repel mosquitos.

Safety: Avoid taking vitex while pregnant or breast-feeding; vitex may inhibit the production of the hormone prolactin, which stimulates the production of breast milk. Skin rashes have been a problem for a low number of women. Most therapies take from three to six months.

Special Instructions: Vitex may interfere with the action of the digestive stimulant Reglan. It also may interfere with certain tranquilizers such as Haldol, Prolixin and Thorazine. If you currently take any of these drugs, consult your physician before starting vitex therapy.

Product Availability: Vitex is available in tablets, capsules, liquid extracts, and as an elixir. It is sometimes combined with other herbs such as black cohosh in combinations designed to treat PMS, menopause, mood disorders and osteoporosis.

Complementary Agents: natural progesterone cream, red clover, soy isoflavones, black cohosh, evening primrose oil

References

Milewicz et al. 1993. Vitex agnus castus extract in the treatment of luteal phase defects due to latent hyperprolactinemia. Results of a randomized placebo-controlled double-blind study. *Arzneimittelforschung* 43(7):752–56.

Schellenberg et al. 2000. Treatment for the premenstrual syndrome with agnus castus fruit extract: prospective, randomized placebo controlled study. *British Medical Journal* 20:322(7279: 134–7).

Tschudin et al. 1999. Treatment of cyclical mastalgia with a solution containing a Vitex agnus castus extract: Results of a placebo-controlled double-blind study. *Breast* 8:175–181.

Watanabe, K. et al. 1995. Rotundial, a new natural mosquito repellent from the leaves of Vitex rotundifolia. *Biosci Biotechnol Biochem* 59(10):1979–80.

Chickweed *(Stellaria media)*

Overview: This small, green annual plant grows across this country and originally came from Europe. It can be found growing in yards and fields everywhere. Herbal practitioners traditionally used it to expel fevers and to soothe breast inflammation. It contains volatile oils that have an antiseptic action used to ease irritations of the gastrointestinal tract and to treat asthma. Today, its main use is found in cream form for treating rashes and other inflammatory skin disorders.

Therapeutic Applications: Topical: cuts, wounds, skin itching and irritation, eczema, psoriasis Internal: rheumatism, ulcers, gout, blood diseases

Scientific Updates: Currently there are no studies on this particular herb.

Safety: Chickweed is considered safe although taking it in large doses is not recommended.

Special Instructions: Chickweed cream preparations can be applied liberally several times daily to treat rashes and inflammatory skin conditions like eczema. As a tincture, 1 to 5 ml daily is commonly used. Chickweed can also be made in to a tea or can be used effectively for skin irritations as a bath additive.

Product Availability: Although Chickweed is still available as a single herbal supplement, it is more commonly used in cream or ointment preparations.

Complementary Agents: aloe vera, calendula, St. John's wort

References

Duke, J.A. 1985. *CRC Handbook of Medicinal Herbs*. Boca Raton: CRC Press. p. 458-9.

Weiss, R.F. 1988. *Herbal Medicine*. Gothenburg, Sweden: Ab Arcanum. p. 265.

Chlorella *(Chlorella pyrenoidosa)*

Overview: Chlorella is a single-celled green algae thought to have the richest content of chlorophyll of any known plant. Chlorella has traditionally been used as a blood detoxifier. Chlorella contains an impressive array of vitamins and minerals including nineteen amino acids, RNA and DNA. Like other forms of algae, it is recommended for boosting the immune system and inhibiting both bowel and blood toxicity.

Therapeutic Applications: weak immune system, high blood pressure, high cholesterol levels, radiation exposure, heavy metal poisoning, chronic fatigue syndrome, peptic ulcers, indigestion, bad breath, constipation, free radical exposure, cancer, cataracts, chronic diseases, chronic fatigue, diabetes, hepatitis, glaucoma, obesity

Scientific Updates: Recent tests are evaluating chlorella's phycocyanin content for cancer treatment. Anecdotal data suggests that marine algae like spirulina and chlorella can help to protect against ultraviolet radiation. Compounds in blue-green algae have also been linked to cholesterol lowering and weight loss. New data suggests that chlorella can also prevent stress-induced peptic ulcers and lowers cancer risk. It may also benefit anyone with fibromyalgia.

Safety: The ability of algae to absorb and even concentrate heavy metals such as lead and mercury from contaminated water is a concern. For this reason, it is not wise to consume more than 50 grams of blue-green algae supplements daily. Excessive intake may also cause gout or kidney stones. If you have a history of either, you should avoid algae products. Scientists have not determined safe doses of chlorella in pregnant and nursing women, young children, and individuals with kidney or liver disease. Some people have reported severe reactions to the supplement. In addition, some chemicals in chlorella may cause photosensitivity (sensitivity to sun exposure) and may interfere with anticlotting medications like warfarin.

Special Instructions: It is vital to obtain any type of blue-green algae from a reliable source to ensure purity. Remember that excess ingestion of chlorella may cause fatigue.

Product Availability: Chlorella can be purchased in powder, juice, extract, liquid concentrate, capsule, soft gel, tablets, or granules.

Complementary Agents: spirulina, chlorophyll, red clover, barley and wheat grass, milk thistle, antioxidant compounds

References

Dantas, D. and M. Queiroz. 1999. Effects of Chlorella vulgaris on bone marrow progenitor cells of mice infected with Listeria monocytogenes. *International Journal of Immunopharmacology* 21(8):499–508.

Lee, R.E. 1989. *Phycology 2nd ed.* Cambridge: Cambridge University Press. p. 91.

Merchant et al. 2000. Nutritional Supplementation with Chlorella pyrenoidosa for patients with fibromyalgia syndrome: a pilot study. *Phytotherapy Research* 14(3):167–73.

Cinnamon *(Cinnamomum ssp.)*

Overview: Cinnamon is a small evergreen tree that is native to Asia and actually encompasses a number of species. The species *Cinnamomum cassia* or simply *cassia* is known as Chinese cinnamon and is used in natural medicine; however, the species *Cinnamomum zeylanicum* is considered the most potent of cinnamon trees. The bark and the oil of cinnamon trees are used to treat digestive complaints and microbial infections, among other things.

Therapeutic Applications: appetite loss, anorexia, gas, bloating, indigestion, intestinal cramps, microbe infections, skin cuts/abrasions, menstrual pain, coughs, colds, sore throat, yeast infections, heavy periods

Scientific Updates: The volatile oils found in cinnamon may help promote better digestion by breaking down fats. Studies show that it stimulates the secretion of bile, which helps expedite the metabolism of food. Cinnamon may also protect against peptic ulcers, act as an appetite stimulant and fight yeast infections. The most active compounds in cinnamon are eugenol and cinnamaldehyde.

Safety: Some people are allergic to cinnamon, especially when they are exposed to a concentrated form, such as the essential oil. Symptoms of cinnamon allergy include asthma and skin irritations. A cinnamon overdose can result in symptoms of increased breathing, fast heartbeat, sweating and even a slow down of the central nervous system. Some individuals develop allergies and dermatitis after exposure to cinnamon. For this reason use only small amounts. Do not use cinnamon if you are pregnant or if you have ulcers.

Special Instructions: Cinnamon tea can be made from the powdered herb by boiling half a teaspoon (2 to 3 grams) of the powder for fifteen minutes. Only a few drops of essential oil should be used and never for extended periods of time. Cinnamon tincture in the amount of 2–3 ml three times each day can also be taken. When using oil of cinnamon, never apply directly to skin or consume in large amounts. Always dilute oil in carrier of some sort.

Product Availability: Cinnamon comes in essential oils, powders, teas, extracts and capsules.

Complementary Agents: cloves, peppermint, fennel, artichoke

References

Akira et al. 1999. Pharmacological studies on the antiulcerogenic activity of Chinese cinnamon. *Planta Medica* 6:440.

Azumi et al. 1997. A novel inhibitor of bacterial endotoxin derived from cinnamon bark. *Biochem Biophys Res Commun* 234:506–10.

Quale et al. 1996. In vitro activity of Cinnamomum zeylanicum against azole resistant and sensitive Candida species and a pilot study of cinnamon for oral candidiasis. *American Journal of Chinese Medicine* 24:103–9.

Singh et al. 1995. Cinnamon bark oil, a potent fungitoxicant against fungi causing respiratory tract mycoses. *Allergy* 50:995–99.

Comfrey *(Symphytum officinale)*

Overview: Comfrey is a much used herb that comes from the roots and leaves of a plant called *Symphytum officinale,* which belongs to the borage family. It is also referred to as "boneset" due to its popular use as a bone mender. It has also been used as a digestive aid and in topical applications to treat wounds and broken bones. Today, however, its internal use is discouraged due to its toxicity. Comfrey aids bone and muscle injuries because it is readily absorbed through the skin.

Therapeutic Applications: burns, wounds, sprains, insect bites, fractures, sores, swelling, pain

Scientific Updates: It is the allantoin content of comfrey that gives it the ability to stimulate new cell growth and cell proliferation, and to alleviate pain. For this reason, topical applications of comfrey are ideal for any type of healing, especially wounds and bone fractures.

Safety: Comfrey should never be taken orally (by mouth) unless by medical prescription and supervision. It can cause significant liver damage. Compounds called pyrrolizidine alkaloids are what make comfrey internal so toxic. The American Herbal Products Association has listed comfrey in its "Restricted Use Category" and only approves it for external use.

Special Instructions: Only use comfrey on the surface of the skin, and follow manufacturer's label instruction.

Product Availability: Comfrey is commonly found in combination products containing aloe vera, witch hazel, arnica or calendula in ointments or creams. You can also purchase comfrey in fresh or dried leaf form or in concentrated drops, extracts and tinctures. Allantoin is also commonly added to skin care products.

Complementary Agents: aloe vera, calendula cream, witch hazel, horse chestnut, arnica

References

Abbott, P.J. 1988. Comfrey: assessing the low-dose health risk. *Medical Journal of Australia* 149(11–12):678–82.

Couet, C.E. 1996. Analysis, separation, and bioassay of pyrrolizidine alkaloids from comfrey (Symphytum officinale). *Natural Toxins* 4(4):163–7.

Cornsilk *(Zea mays)*

Overview: Cornsilk refers to the soft, hair-like growth found in an ear of corn or maize. This fine silk is usually collected when the corn is in milk and is used when still green. Cornsilk compounds, which include maizenic acid, act as cardiac tonics and diuretics. The Incas used cornsilk as a treatment for urogenital infections, and by 1800, it was marketed in Europe by Parke-Davis.

Therapeutic Applications: albuminuria, bladder infections, edema, heart trouble, hepatitis, kidney disorders, prostatitis, urinary tract infections, water retention

Scientific Updates: The maizenic acid contained in cornsilk is responsible for its stimulating diuretic effect. In addition, this compound also benefits the liver and intestines and is considered a cardiac tonic for the heart. Clinical studies in China and Japan have demonstrated cornsilk's remarkable diuretic properties. Cornsilk directly reduces painful symptoms and swelling caused by inflammatory conditions such as cystitis, pyelitis, oliguria, and hepatitis. In China, it is also used for hypertension and diabetes.

Safety: Cornsilk is considered a mild, nontoxic herb. Take in appropriate doses as directed. Any substance that acts as a diuretic may cause a potassium deficiency if used in excess. Do not take cornsilk if you are taking any other diuretic preparations or if you have kidney disease or high blood pressure.

Special Instructions: When taking cornsilk or any other natural diuretic, make sure to drink plenty of pure water.

Product Availability: Cornsilk can be purchased as a single herb but is also commonly found in combinations designed to support the urinary system that may include cranberry, buchu, parsley and uva ursi.

Complementary Agents: buchu, parsley, uva ursi, cranberry, juniper berries, marshmallow, couch grass, vitamin C, bioflavonoids, proanthocyanidins, B-complex, vitamin E, magnesium, potassium, copper, mineral and electrolyte supplements

References

Leung, A.Y. 1984. *Chinese Herbal Remedies.* New York: Universe Books. p. 47–49.

Mowrey, Daniel B. 1986. *The Scientific Validation of Herbal Medicine. Keats Publishing.* Connecticut: Keats. p. 2.

Couch Grass *(Agropyron repens)*

Overview: Couch grass has a natural diuretic action, which makes it an ideal treatment for any type of urinary tract infection. Couch grass can stimulate urine discharge and may help to pass kidney stones. It is also considered a demulcent, which works to heal irritated mucous membranes in the case of urinary tract infections.

Therapeutic Applications: bladder infections, blood purifier, jaundice, kidney disease, kidney stones, rheumatism

Scientific Update: Couch grass contains mannitol, which acts not only as a natural diuretic, but is also a healing mucilage. The mannitol contained in this herb also has a mild antibiotic effects on a variety of bacteria and molds. Couch grass may help to eliminate kidney stones.

Safety: Take in appropriate doses as recommended. An excess could lead to potassium and other mineral deficiencies.

Special Instructions: Couch grass can be taken as an infusion (tea) or in tincture form.

Product Availability: Couch grass is available in capsules, tinctures and extracts. It is often added to urinary tract formulas containing juniper berries or buchu, which works to potentiates its antibiotic action.

Complementary Agents: uva ursi, juniper berries, cornsilk, parsley, juniper, cascara sagrada, red clover, garlic, , vitamin C, bioflavonoids, vitamin A, vitamin E, potassium

References

Ody, Penelope. 1993. *The Complete Medicinal Herbal.* Dorling-Kinderseley. p. 158.

Ritchason, Jack. 1994. *The Little Herb Encyclopedia. 3rd ed.* Pleasant Grove, Utah: Woodland Books. p. 63–64.

Cramp Bark *(Viburnum opulus)*

Overview: Known since the 14th century, cramp bark was used by American Indians to treat the mumps and other conditions that cause swelling. Cramp bark is most famous for its ability to relax the uterus and has traditionally been used by folk practitioners to treat menstrual cramps, muscle spasms, and abdominal cramps. It is also good for heart muscle and exerts a calming effect in cases of hysteria or nervousness.

Therapeutic Applications: asthma, colic, constipation, digestive disorders, edema, menstrual cramps, muscle cramps, heart disorders, hypertension, hysteria, leg cramps, nervousness, uterine cramps, afterbirth pains

Scientific Updates: Cramp bark is a potent muscle relaxant that exerts a very specific action on the uterus and is considered a good herbal remedy for menstrual pain. This herb has been recognized in the *National Formulary* as a specific antispasmodic also useful for attacks of asthma and hysteria. Studies also suggest that it potentiates the ability of cardiac muscle to pump blood.

Safety: Pregnant or nursing women should not use this herb. Cramp bark should not be combined with any blood thinning drugs.

Special Instructions: Tinctures seem to work more readily for muscle pain and menstrual cramps, and should be used according to label instructions.

Product Availability: Apart from being available in standard capsules, extracts, teas, etc., cramp bark can be purchased in cream or ointment from for direct application to sore muscles.

Complementary Agents: squaw vine, dong quai, damiana, red raspberry, licorice, sarsaparilla, black cohosh, wild yam, peppermint, valerian root, niacin vitamin E, vitamin C, bioflavonoids, folic acid, calcium/magnesium

References

Calle et al. 1999. Antinociceptive and uterine relaxant activities of Viburnum toronis alive (Caprifoliaceae). *Journal of Ethnopharmacology* 66(1):71–3.

Digitalis-type cardiotonic action of Viburnum species extracts. 1977. *Planta Medica* 31(3):228–31.

Ody, Penelope. 1993. *The Complete Medicinal Herbal.* Dorling-Kinderseley. p. 113.

Cranberry (Vaccinium macrocarpon)

Overview: Cranberries have been used both in culinary dishes and in medicinal applications. Native to North America, the use of the whole berry in dried extracts has become much more popular. Used to prevent and treat urinary tract infections, the therapeutic compounds found in cranberry are relatively new to science. Past practitioners also used the herb to treat stomach disorders and gallbladder disease. Cranberry is rich in vitamin C and flavonoids (proanthocyanidins), which are powerful antioxidant agents.

Therapeutic Applications: bladder infections, urinary tract infections, high cholesterol, prostatitis

Scientific Updates: A 1994 study published in the *Journal of the American Medical Association* found that ten ounces per day of a commercially available cranberry juice cocktail was almost twice as effective as a placebo in reducing bacteria in urine. Although cranberry juice may turn urine more acidic, it makes infections less likely. Recent data shows that compounds in cranberry prevent bacteria like *E. coli* from sticking to the lining of the bladder and urinary tract. Cranberry may also benefit cholesterol levels and has anticancer properties as well.

Safety: Do not take cranberry if your are on drugs for a urinary tract infection or for kidney problems. Cranberry can be taken during pregnancy and breastfeeding.

Special Instructions: If you are fighting or trying to prevent recurring urinary tract infections, drink both the pure juice and take the whole cranberry in capsule form as directed. Several glasses (16 ounces) of a concentrated juice product can approximate the effect of the cranberry concentrate. Cranberry tincture, in the amount of 3 to 5 ml three times per day can also be taken.

Product Availability: Look for products that contain dried, unsweetened juice, powder or concentrated extract. Some products add vitamin C and flavonoids. You may also drink unsweetened pure cranberry juice, which is quite bitter and often difficult to find. Sweetened cranberry juice products may be easier to drink but should contain 30 percent or more pure cranberry juice.

Complementary Agents: burdock, uva ursi, juniper berry, goldenrod, goldenseal, alfalfa, cornsilk, vitamin C, bioflavonoids, proanthocyanidins, vitamin A, zinc

References

Ahuja et al. 1998. Loss of fimbrial adhesion with the addition of Vaccinum macrocarpon to the growth medium of P-fimbriated Escherichia coli. *Journal of Urology* 159(2):559–62.

Avorn et al. 1994. Reduction of bacteriuria and pyuria after ingestion of cranberry juice. *Journal of the American Medical Association* 271:751.

Bomser et al. 1996. In-vitro anticancer activity of fruit extracts from Vaccinium species. *Planta Medica* 62(3):212–16.

Wilson et al. 1998. Cranberry extract inhibits low density lipoprotein oxidation. *Life Science* 62(24):PL381–86.

Culver's Root (*Veronicastrum virgincum*)

Overview: Used for generations by Native Americans, this herb helps expel old debris from the bowel, boosts liver function, clears congestion and is considered a natural relaxant. Culver's root contains a number of phytochemicals that have been used in folk medicine. It was named after Dr. Coulvert, an American physician who practiced in the early 18th century. It is considered an old-fashioned American remedy for liver congestion and constipation.

Therapeutic Applications: constipation, diarrhea, colon congestion, liver ailments, stomach disorders, blood purifier

Scientific Updates: Culver's root works chiefly on the intestines in cases of chronic constipation due to poor biliary flow. It has a mild action without causing the weakness that can be seen with other purgative medicines. Leptandrin, a compound found in culver's root, stimulates the liver and promotes the secretion of bile without irritating the bowels.

Safety: Pregnant or nursing mothers should not take this herb without their doctor's consent. Taking fennel or ginger with this herb helps to prevent the formation of intestinal gas.

Special Instructions: Combining culver's root with other natural laxatives such as cascara sagrada enhances its actions. You may also want to add ginger in supplemental form to prevent flatulence.

Product Availability: Culver's root is available in capsules, tinctures, extracts and teas.

Complementary Agents: buckthorn, cascara sagrada, red raspberry, ginger, fennel, black walnut, quassia, garlic, couch grass, acidophilus, vitamin C, bioflavonoids, vitamin A, B-complex, marine lipids, blue-green algae

References

Grieve M. A. 1994. *Modern Herbal.* New York: Dorset.

Hutchens, Alma. 1969. *Indian Herbology of North America.* Ontario, Canada:Merco. p. 108.

Damiana *(Tunera aphrodisiaca)*

Overview: Utilized as medicines by the indigenous cultures of Central America, damiana was primarily used for treating female disorders. It was also considered a sexual restorative, a remedy for menopause, and a reproductive system tonic. Damiana also has chemical constituents that stimulate the central nervous system and was used by Mexican folk practitioners to treat asthma and bronchitis.

Therapeutic Applications: aphrodisiac, impotence, depression, fatigue, female problems, hormonal imbalances, infertility, menopause, mood swings, Parkinson's disease, PMS, prostate disorders, sexual dysfunction

Scientific Updates: There is some evidence that damiana benefits sexual debility and nervous tension. Damiana has also been used as a stimulating nervine tonic to treat depression. It has been applied in cases of chronic fatigue and mental exhaustion and contains beta-sitosterol, which may explain its positive effect on the reproductive system. It has been used for both male and female infertility.

Special Instructions: For damiana tea, add 1 cup boiling water to 1 gram of dried leaves and steep for fifteen minutes. Drink three cups daily. In tincture form, take 2–3 ml three times daily. Tablets or capsules are commonly taken in 400 to 800 mg doses three times daily.

Product Availability: Although this herb is available as a single supplement, it works more effectively when combined with other herbs that have similar therapeutic properties.

Safety: High doses of damiana may create euphoric sensations. Some cases of diarrhea have also been reported.

Complementary Agents: saw palmetto, ginseng, suma, sarsaparilla, dong quai, red raspberry, licorice, kelp, black cohosh, cramp bark, queen of the meadow, ginseng, squaw vine, gotu kola, vitamin E, bee pollen, bee propolis, B-complex, calcium/magnesium, marine lipids

References

Curtin, L. 1965. *Healing Herbs of the Upper Rio Grande.* Los Angeles: Southwest Museum.

Duke, J.A. 1985. *CRC Handbook of Medicinal Herbs.* Boca Raton, FL: CRC Press. p. 492.

Hutchens, Alma. 1969. *Indian Herbology of North America*. Ontario, Canada: Merco. p. 108.

Mills, S.Y. 1991. *Out of the Earth: The Essential Book of Herbal Medicine*. Middlesex, UK: Viking Arkana. p. 516-7.

Dandelion *(Taraxacum officinale)*

Overview: The yellow flowers of the dandelion plant are rich in potassium and work to detoxify the blood, increase the flow of bile from the liver, build red blood cells, and are considered a highly nutritive food. Traditionally the herb has been used as a digestive tonic, blood cleanser, and as mild diuretic and laxative.

Therapeutic Applications: acne, anemia, arthritis, asthma, blood disorders, eczema, gallbladder disease, hepatitis, hypoglycemia, high cholesterol, jaundice, kidney infections, liver disorders, psoriasis, PMS, skin eruptions, weight loss

Scientific Updates: Dandelion leaves are rich in beta-carotene, vitamin C and potassium. Several clinical studies have supported the ability of dandelion to treat chronic liver congestion. Dandelion has an impressive bile-stimulating action, which helps promote liver and gallbladder function. It can also stimulate the elimination of uric acid from the body and helps to stabilize blood sugar.

Safety: Virtually every part of the dandelion plant is edible and considered non-toxic. It may initiate an allergic reaction in certain sensitive individuals, and the leaf and root should not be used by people with gallstones or bile duct obstruction. Anyone with stomach ulcers or gastritis should use dandelion only with their doctor's permission.

Special Instructions: Dandelion in tea form has traditionally been used to purify the blood after infection or as a spring tonic. Taking it in capsule form at a stronger potency is recommended for liver problems or more serious conditions.

Product Availability: Dandelion is available in tablets, capsules, concentrated drops, tinctures, and extracts, and also as a tea.

Complementary Agents: milk thistle, burdock, yellow dock, cascara sagrada, fenugreek, garlic, red sage, red clover, black cohosh, vitamin C, bioflavonoids, proanthocyanidins, vitamin A, B-complex, vitamin E

References

Ingber A. 2000. Seasonal allergic contact dermatitis from Taraxacum officinale (dandelion) in an Israeli florist. *Contact Dermatitis* 43(1):49.

Murray, Michael N.D., and Joseph Pizzorno, N.D. 1991. *Encyclopedia of Natural Medicine.* Rocklin, CA: Prima.

Williams et al. 1996. Flavonoids, cinnamic acids and coumarins from the different tissues and medicinal preparations of Taraxacum officinale. *Phytochemistry* 42(1):121–7.

Devil's Claw *(Harpagophytum procumbens)*

Overview: Devil's claw grows naturally in Southern Africa and the island of Madagascar. Its unique hook-covered fruit prompted its name. Its medicinal value is primarily concentrated in its roots and has been used to treat rheumatism, arthritis and gout by native peoples. Its glycoside content makes it a natural anti-inflammatory agent. Devil's claw is also considered an anti-aging botanical and a vascular tonic. It is an ideal herbal for most geriatric applications.

Therapeutic Applications: arteriosclerosis, arthritis, blood purifier, cholesterol inflammation, edema, indigestion, liver ailments, neuralgia, rheumatism, stomach ailments.

Scientific Updates: Recent studies support Devil's Claw's anti-inflammatory action. In fact, some studies compare it to phenylbutazone, a commonly prescribed drug for arthritis. Harpagoside and other iridoid glycosides and saponins found in devil's claw may be responsible for its anti-inflammatory and analgesic effect. All research, however, does not support its use for arthritis. There is some evidence that it may also help to regulate cholesterol levels. Devil's claw is a potent bitter, containing iridoid glycosides that stimulate stomach secretions, which enhance digestion.

Safety: Extensive data supports the safety of this herb, but it should not be used during pregnancy as it may stimulate uterine contraction. Because it may increase stomach acid, it should not be used by people with gastric or duodenal ulcers.

Special Instructions: It is thought that powdered forms of this herb are more effective as digestive tonics. For tinctures, the recommended dose is 1 to 2 ml per day. If you have arthritis, you may want to try a stronger dose. Consult your health care practitioner.

Product Availability: Devil's claw is often added to joint formulas that contain other natural anti-inflammatory agents and compounds like glucosamine and chondroitin, which help to regenerate cartilage.

Complementary Agents: celery, wild yam, black cohosh, Oregon grape, ginger, glucosamine, chondroitin, vitamin C, bioflavonoids, grapeseed or pine bark extract, essential fatty acids

References

Grahame, R. and B.V. Robinson. 1981. Devil's claw (Harpogophytum procumbens): pharmacological and clinical studies. *Ann Rheum Dis* 40:632.

Leung, A.Y. and S. Foster. 1996. *Encyclopedia of Common Natural Ingredients Used in Food, Drugs, and Cosmetics, 2nd ed.* New York: John Wiley & Sons. p. 208-10.

Murray, Michael N.D., and Joseph Pizzorno, N.D. 1991. *Encyclopedia of Natural Medicine.* Rocklin, CA: Prima.

Tyler, V.E. 1993. *The Honest Herbal. 3d ed.* Binghamton, NY: Pharmaceutical Products Press: 111-12.

Dong Quai *(Angelica sinensis)*

Overview: A member of the celery family and considered one of the best herbal uterine tonics, dong quai is very highly regarded by oriental medical practitioners. Known as the female ginseng, it has been used to correct painful menstruation, hormonal imbalance, postpartum conditions, and menopausal symptoms. It also has a good track record for high blood pressure and disorders of peripheral circulation.

Therapeutic Applications: atherosclerosis, fatigue, high blood pressure, Reynaud's disease, hormonal imbalance, menstrual disorders, menopause, fibrocystic breast disease, muscle spasms

Scientific Updates: The chemical constituents of dong quai have an immediate stimulatory effect on the uterus. This herb strengthens and normalizes uterine contractions. Both animal and human studies have found that dong quai improves peripheral circulation. Research indicates that it is the ferulic acid and lulgustilide content of the herb that prevents spasms and relaxes blood vessels.

Safety: Dong quai has no reported toxicity. It should be avoided in cases of severe gastrointestinal disease and should not be used by pregnant or nursing women. This herb should not be used by anyone with hemorrhagic diseases and should be avoided during severe cases of the flu or in cases of spontaneous abortion. It may also cause fair-skinned people to become more sensitive to sunlight.

Special Instructions: While it is common for women to take up to 4 grams daily, consult with your health care practitioner to determine the appropriate dose for your situation.

Product Availability: Powdered root supplements are available in capsules, tablets, tinctures or teas.

Complementary Agents: black cohosh, cramp bark, squaw vine, queen of the meadow, sarsaparilla, licorice, damiana, red raspberry, saw palmetto, wild yam, vitamin E, vitamin C, bioflavonoids, B-complex, calcium/magnesium, evening primrose oil

References

Flynn, Rebecca M.S., and Mark Roest. 1995. *Your Guide to Standardized Herbal Products*. Prescott AZ: One World. p. 4.

Foster, S. and Y. Chongxi. 1992. *Herbal Emissaries*. Rochester, VT: Healing Arts Press. p. 65–72.

Qi-bing et al. 1991. Advances in the pharmacological studies of radix Angelica sinensis (Oliv) Diels (Chinese danggui). *Chinese Medical Journal* 104:776–81.

Echinacea *(Echinacea purpurea)*

Overview: Echinacea is a very popular herb and comes from the purple coneflower *(Echinacea angustifolia, E. purpurea, E. pallida)*, which grows wild in North America. Used extensively by Native American people, echinacea was used to treat snakebites and wounds. Because it has natural antibiotic actions, echinacea is considered an excellent herb for infections of all kinds. In addition, it works to boost lymphatic cleansing of the blood and enhances the immune system. It also has natural cortisone-like properties, which contribute to its anti-inflammatory action.

Therapeutic Applications: acne, arthritis, blood cleansing, boils, burns, bronchitis, canker sores, chronic fatigue, colds, congestion, contagious diseases, ear infections, fevers, herpes, glandular disorders, infections (viral and bacterial), influenza, immune system disorders, prostate disease, psoriasis, tonsillitis, wounds, yeast infections

Scientific Updates: Laboratory tests have discovered that compounds found in echinacea have the ability to recognize and rearrange enzyme patterns in the body. The ability of this herb to boost immune function deals with thymus gland stimulation. Echinacea can actually stimulate the production and action of interferon and natural killer cells. It may also help the body neutralize carcinogenic substances. There is substantial clinical evidence that sufficient oral doses of echinacea can reduce the duration and severity of upper respiratory infections. Data from two placebo-controlled, double-blind German studies indicate that therapeutic doses of *Echinacea purpurea* may reduce the severity of colds, and that continuous use may reduce their frequency. Other studies show that echinacea may be effective in suppressing yeast infections. When applied externally to cuts, bites, stings, abrasions, etc, echinacea helps promote tissue healing and inhibits inflammation. In one study of 4,598 patients with various skin conditions, a topical *E. purpurea* ointment was effective in treating over 85 percent of test subjects with wounds, burns, eczema, varicose ulcers and herpes. New data also suggests that echinacea may help to inhibit leukemia.

Safety: One of the least toxic herbs, echinacea is not known to cause any side effects when taken orally. Allergic reactions are rare but can be life threatening in certain individuals. You may want to try a very small dose at first if you're allergic to other plants in the ragweed family. If you have an autoimmune illness, such as lupus, or other progressive disease such as multiple sclerosis, consult with a physician before taking echinacea. There are no known contraindications to the use of echinacea during pregnancy or breast-feeding. High doses of echinacea may occasionally cause nausea and dizziness. Anyone suffering from any type of kidney disorder should not take echinacea for longer than one-week intervals due to the possible excretion of minerals. Heavy or prolonged use of this herb is not recommended.

Special Instructions: One German study indicates that echinacea's immune-stimulating effects begin to subside after five days. In addition, as a general immune stimulant, most herbalists recommend that you stop taking echinacea for a week after six or eight weeks of continuous use.

Product Availability: Echinacea is available in a wide variety of dry and liquid forms, including freeze-dried, tablets, juice, capsules, concentrated drops, tinctures, teas, ointments, creams, and gels. Echinacea extracts are often standardized to certain percentages of echinacosides. Echinacea is frequently combined with goldenseal, elderberry, vitamin C, zinc, bee propolis, olive leaf, vitamin A, etc. There is some speculation that the potency of liquid echinacea extract is linked to the tingling sensation it creates on the tongue; however, this has not been scientifically documented.

Complementary Agents: cat's claw, cordyceps, goldenseal, pau d'arco, astragalus, olive leaf, garlic, transfer factor, elderberry, vitamin C, bioflavonoids, vitamin A, blue-green algae, B-complex vitamins, vitamin A, calcium-magnesium, zinc

References

Braunig et al. 1992. Echinacea: Clinical trial re: rhinovirus. *Zeitschrift fur Phytotherapie* 13:7.

Coeugniet et al. 1986. Echinacea: Clinical trial re: Candiasis. *Therapiewoche* 36:3352.

Currier, N. and S. Miller 2000. Natural killer cells from aging mice treated with extracts from Echinacea purpurea are quantitatively and functionally rejuvenated. *Experimental Gerontology* 35(5):627–39.

Facino et al. 1995. Echinacoside and caffeoyl conjugates protect collagen from free radical-induced degradation: A potential use of Echinacea extracts in the prevention of skin photodamage. *Planta Medica* 61:510–14.

Hayashi et al. 2001. Effects of oral administration of Echinacea purpurea (American herb) on incidence of spontaneous leukemia caused by recombinant leukemia viruses in AKR/J mice. *Nihon Rinsho Meneki Gakkai Kaishi* 24(1):10–20.

Jurcic et al. 1989. Echinacea: duration of effect. *Zeitschrift fur Phytotherapie* 10:67–70.

Melchart et al. 1998. Echinacea: Clinical trial re: rhinovirus. *Archives of Family Medicine.* Nov–Dec.

Melchart et al. 1995. Results of five randomized studies on the immunomodulatory activity of preparations of Echinacea. *Alternative and Complementary Medicine* 1(2):145–60.

Elderberry *(Sambucus nigra)*

Overview: Elderberry grows wild in parts of Europe and North America. Both the dark purple berry and light flowers of the elder shrub are used medicinally. Traditionally, the plant was utilized in topical remedies for skin and mouth ailments and internally to induce sweating and relieve constipation. Elderberry pie is a popular dish.

New scientific data now supports the ability of elderberry to shorten the duration of certain viral infections.

Therapeutic Applications: colds, flu, sore throat, herpes infections, chronic fatigue, muscle and joint pain (from inflammation)

Scientific Updates: According to laboratory research, an extract from the leaves, combined with St. John's wort and soapwort, inhibits the influenza virus and herpes simplex virus. Israeli scientists tested a standardized extract of the berry on forty people and found that it prompted significant improvement in flu symptoms or even caused test subjects to become cured in almost 90 percent of cases in two to three days compared to six days for a control group. In another study, an elderberry extract was considered an effective treatment for influenza, and other trials have shown its anti-inflammatory activity.

Safety: While the berry product is considered safe when taken orally, any product made from the leaves or bark of the elderberry tree should not be taken internally.

Special Instructions: Liquid extracts are typically used in doses from 5 ml twice daily for children to 10 ml twice daily for adults. You can also make elderberry tea by steeping 5 grams of the dried flowers in 1 cup of boiling water for fifteen minutes taken three times daily.

Product Availability: Elderberry can be purchased in tinctures, liquid extracts, lozenges, syrups, standardized extract capsules, throat sprays and concentrated drops.

Complementary Agents: echinacea, goldenseal, olive leaf, garlic, cat's claw, pau d'arco, zinc, vitamin A, vitamin C, transfer factor

References:
Mascolo et al. 1987. Biological screening of Italian medicinal plants for anti-inflammatory activity. *Phytotherapy Research* 1:28–31.

Serkedjieva et al. 1990. Antiviral activity of the infusion (SHS-174) from flowers of Sambucus nigra L., aerial parts of Hypericum perforatum L., and roots of Saponaria officinalis L. against influenza and herpes simplex viruses. *Phytotherapy Research* 4:97–100.

Zakay-Rones et al. 1995. Inhibition of several strains of influenza virus in vitro and reduction of symptoms by an elderberry extract (Sambucus nigra L.) during an outbreak of influenza B in Panama. *Journal of Alternative and Complementary Medicine* 1,4:361–69.

Ephedra *(Ephedra sinica)*

Overview: Ephedra in its various forms has been used for millennia both in eastern and western cultures. There are over thrity varieties of ephedra from the North American species, called Mormon tea (*Ephedra nevadensis*), to the more popular Chinese form, also known as *ma huang (Ephedra sinica)*. Mormon tea or *Ephedra nevadensis* does not contain the alkaloids that give ma haung its medicinal effects and potential risks. Traditional Chinese practitioners used ma huang *(Ephedra sinica)* to treat bronchial spasms typically seen in asthma attacks. Synthetic ephedrine compounds are commonly included in over-the-counter cold remedies. Recent controversy surrounding ephedra deals with its overuse for weight loss, potential health risks and abuse by young people.

Therapeutic Applications: some types of asthma, nasal congestion, some allergies, obesity

Scientific Updates: Chinese ephedra contains an adrenaline-like compound called ephedrine, which stimulates the central nervous system, elevates blood pressure, increases heart rate and causes the body to lose fluids. Several studies indicate that ephedra does indeed dilate bronchiole tubes and helps with nasal congestion. It has also been found to aid in the conversion of fat to heat when mixed with other compounds. Other studies suggest that it may be of benefit for people with inflammatory autoimmune diseases.

Special Instructions: The maximum recommended dosage of ephedrine for a healthy adult is between 100 to 300 mg per day, taken in equal doses of no more than 30 mg each. Do not take ephedra for extended periods of time. Children should not be given this herb unless under a doctor's supervision. It is not intended for anyone under eighteen. If you are using it for weight loss, do not assume that more is better. Overdosing on ephedra can be life threatening.

Product Availability: Ephedra is sold dried and in capsules, concentrated drops, tinctures, and extracts. It is often the main component of weight loss formulas designed to speed up the metabolism. Make sure you are not taking it as a single supplement and in a combination simultaneously.

Safety: While ephedra has been used safely for millennia, abusing this herb can be very dangerous. Excessive amounts of ephedra can cause heart attacks, heart arrhythmias, seizures, strokes or even death. Recent studies show that up to half of people who take ephedra experience elevated heart rates, which can also occur when taking over-the-counter products containing ephedrine. Always check with your doctor before taking ephedra and avoid the herb if you have high blood pressure, heart or thyroid disease, diabetes, prostate enlargement or urinary tract problems. Do not use ephedra if you are pregnant or nursing or have anxiety, anorexia, bulimia, glaucoma, cerebral perfusions, pheochromocytoma or thyrotoxicosis. If you feel nervous, have tremors, insomnia, appetite loss or nausea, discontinue use. Be aware that prolonged use of ephedra is not recommended since it can compromise the adrenal glands. Do not use ephedra-containing products if you are taking a MAO inhibitor or any other prescription drug. Even though it has stimulant effects, ephedra can make you drowsy, so use it with caution if you are driving or operating machinery.

Complementary Agents: *Garcinia cambogia,* white willow bark, vitamin C with bioflavonoids

References

Astrup et al. 1992. The effect of ephedrine/caffeine mixture on energy expenditure and body composition in obese women. *Metabolism* 41(7):686–88.

Blumenthal, M. and P. King. 1995. Ma huang: Ancient herb, modern medicine, regulatory dilemma: A review of the botany, chemistry, medicinal uses, safety concerns, and legal status of ephedra and its alkaloids. *HerbalGram* 34:22–57.

Chase, S.L. 2001. Ephedra is linked to CNS, cardiovascular risks. *RN* 64(2):103.

Ephedra dangers documented. 2000. *Health News* Dec. 6(12):6.

Gurley et al. 2000. Content versus label claims in ephedra-containing dietary supplements. *American Journal of Health System Pharmacology* 15:57(10):963–9.

Eyebright *(Euphrasia officinalis)*

Overview: For generations, eyebright has been a favorite choice for the treatment of various eye diseases. It is particularly effective for any inflammation of the mucous membrane of the eye, as well as for sensitivity to light, minor eye irritations, weeping, itching, etc. Eyebright is grown commercially in Europe where the whole plant herb is used in medicinal products. Traditional uses included making a poultice for eye inflammations such as blepharitis and sties. It was also used for eye fatigue and vision problems. Other uses include respiratory tract infections.

Therapeutic Applications: allergic reactions (eye-related), cataracts, conjunctivitis, irritated eyes, diabetic retinopathy, eye inflammations, eye infections, eyestrain, glaucoma, vision problems

Safety: Eyebright has astringent compounds, which explain its benefit for inflamed eyes. Be aware that the sterility of all applications of eyebright is of utmost concern. Using any substance directly in the eye can cause bacterial infection. There is very little scientific data on the topical use of this herb. Internal use is considered generally safe; however, its safety in pregnant or nursing women has not been established.

Special Instructions: A compress can be made from a decoction of eyebright and the tea can also be taken internally as well. Boil 10 to 15 grams of the dried herb in 4 cups of water for fifteen minutes. You can soak a cotton cloth with the tea and use it as a compress after it cools. You can also take it as a tea two to three times daily. The tincture is typically taken internally in 2 to 5 ml doses three times per day.

Product Availability: Eyebright can be purchased in loose dried form, as a tea, capsulized supplement, tincture or extract. It may also be found as an ingredient in some natural eye products.

Complementary Agents: bilberry, red raspberry, goldenseal, grape seed or pine bark extract, vitamin A, beta-carotene, vitamin C, bioflavonoids

References
Commission E. Monograph. 1992. Euphrasia, Bundesanzeiger.

Hoffman, D. 1988. *The Herbal Handbook: A User's Guide to Medical Herbalism.* Rochester, VT: Healing Arts Press.

Ody, Penelope. 1993. *The Complete Medicinal Herbal.* New York: Dorling-Kinderesley. p. 140-41.

Wichtl, M. 1994. *Herbal Drugs and Phytopharmaceuticals.* Boca Raton, FL: CRC Press. p. 195-6.

False Unicorn (*Chamaelirium luteum*)

Overview: This herb grows wild in parts of Mississippi and the American south. Used by Native Americans primarily for women's health concerns, it was recommended for miscarriage, lack of periods, heavy and painful menstruation and morning sickness. It is the roots of this plant that contain its therapeutic compounds.

Therapeutic Applications: amenorrhea, heavy or painful periods, PMS, menopause

Scientific Updates: The steroidal saponins found in false unicorn are thought to give it an estrogenic action although lack of scientific inquiry does not support this assumption. Traditional herbalists believe that it can stimulate the ovaries after a hysterectomy or post menopause.

Special Instructions: Typically false unicorn root is taken in tincture form at 2 to 4 ml daily.

Product Availability: You will find that false unicorn is rarely taken as a singular herb and is commonly added to female formulas. Some herbalists feel that it is more effective when taken in tincture form.

Safety: The herb is thought to be generally safe; and although it was used by pregnant women in traditional applications, science has not established its safety for pregnant or nursing women.

Complementary Agents: vitex (*Vitex agnus-castus*), soy isoflavones, natural progesterone cream, red clover, black cohosh, wild yam

References

Mills, S.Y. 1991. *Out of the Earth: The Essential Book of Herbal Medicine.* Middlesex, UK: Viking Arkana. p. 520–22.

Ody, Penelope. 1993. *The Complete Medicinal Herbal.* New York: Dorling-Kinderesley. p. 140–41.

Fennel (*Foeniculum vulgare*)

Overview: Used as an effective carminative for digestive problems, fennel relieves intestinal gas and colic. In fact it was added to several European dishes not only for flavor, but to boost digestion as well. Fennel promotes the expulsion of mucus, stimulates lactation, and has been used for weight loss. Its licorice-like taste makes it a good flavoring agent, enhancing the palatability of other herbal medicines. The plant originally came from Europe.

Therapeutic Applications: appetite suppressant, colic, gas, indigestion, heartburn, intestinal disorders, lactation booster, morning sickness, nausea, sedative (juvenile), uric acid (gout), weight loss, irritable bowel syndrome

Scientific Updates: Recent studies have looked at the estrogenic action of fennel. Its flavonoid content is thought to be responsible for its ability to stop stomach spasms typically seen in colic. The main active constituent of fennel is called terpenoid anethole, which may also be responsible for its estrogenic effect. Recent data shows that this herb also exhibits diuretic, choleretic, analgesic, fever reducing and antimicrobial properties.

Safety: Fennel is generally considered safe, although pregnant or nursing women or women with estrogen driven diseases, (especially cancer) should avoid fennel in large doses due to its estrogenic properties.

Special Instructions: You may chew whole fennel seed after a meal or take it in tea form. For tea, boil 2 to 3 grams of crushed seeds in 1 cup of water for fifteen minutes. Cool the liquid, strain, and then drink three cups daily. In tincture form, 2 to 4 ml can be taken three times daily. Do not give fennel to a child under two without your doctor's approval.

Product Availability: Fennel is often added to digestive formulas and can also be purchased as seeds, tea, capsules, tincture and extracts. You may also find it in chewing gums containing digestive enzymes.

Complementary Agents: catnip, chamomile, ginger, papaya, peppermint, licorice, dandelion, fenugreek, thyme, digestive enzymes, calcium/magnesium, acidophilus, bioflavonoids

References

Duke, J.A. 1985. *CRC Handbook of Medicinal Herbs.* Boca Raton, FL: CRC Press. p. 145–6.

Mowrey, Daniel B. Ph.D. 1986. *The Scientific Validation of Herbal Medicine.* Connecticut: Keats Publishing. p. 2.

Tanira et al. 1996. Pharmacological and toxicological investigations on Foeniculum vulgare dried fruit extract in experimental animals. *Phytotherapy Research* 10:33–6.

Fenugreek *(Trigonella foenum-graecum)*

Overview: Esteemed by the Greeks and Romans, fenugreek was used as a flavoring agent and aphrodisiac. Today it is commonly used to break up and expel mucus, to sooth the gastrointestinal tract and to stimulate milk production. Today, the fenugreek seed is widely used in medicinal applications. Traditional Chinese herbalists used it for kidney problems and ailments of the male reproductive tract. Fenugreek is still enjoyed as a spice in many parts of the world.

Therapeutic Applications: allergies, bronchitis, cholesterol levels, coughs, diabetes, digestive ailments, emphysema, intestinal gas, headache, lung infections, mucus congestion, skin eruptions, atherosclerosis, constipation, high cholesterol, high triglycerides

Scientific Updates: Fenugreek is currently being used to treat diabetes in countries of the Middle East. Because it contains up to 30 percent mucilage, fenugreek works as an effective anti-inflammatory agent and can heal abscesses and other skin eruptions. Steroidal saponins account for many of the beneficial effects of fenugreek, especially when it comes to lowering blood fats. Clinical tests have shown that fenugreek also significantly reduces blood glucose and cholesterol levels in test animals. Fenugreek seeds, which contain diosgenin, may also help to tone uterine muscle and stimulate lactation in nursing mothers. French scientists have found that fenugreek stimulates pancreatic secretion, which enhances digestion.

Safety: Fenugreek should be avoided in pregnancy as it is a uterine stimulant. Diabetics should check with their doctor before using fenugreek for blood sugar control. Large doses can cause intestinal upset and nausea.

Special Instructions: Typical doses of fenugreek range from 5 to 10 grams taken with each meal. As a tincture, 1 to 2 ml of fenugreek can be taken up to three times per day, however the taste is extremely bitter.

Product Availability: Fenugreek seeds are very bitter therefore debitterized seeds or encapsulated products are easier to take.

Complementary Agents: dandelion, myrrh, red clover, lobelia, cornsilk, garlic, yellow dock, goldenseal, vitamin C, bioflavonoids, proanthocyanidins, phytonutrients, blue-green algae, vitamin A, B-complex, chromium

References

Ribes et al. 1986. Antidiabetic effects of subfractions from fenugreek seeds in diabetic dogs. *Proc Soc Exp Biol Med* 182:159–66.

Ribes et al. 1984. Effects of fenugreek seeds on endocrine pancreatic secretions in dogs. *Annals of Nutrition and Metabolism* 28:37–43.

Sauvaire et al. 1991. Implication of steroid saponins and sapogenins in the hypocholesterolemic effect of fenugreek. *Lipids* 26:191–7.

Valette et al. 1984. Hypocholesterolemic effect of fenugreek seed in dogs. *Atherosclerosis* 50:105–111.

Feverfew *(Tanacetum parthenium)*

Overview: Feverfew has received a great deal of publicity over its ability to manage migraine headaches. Traditionally, it was used to bring down a fever and for minor headaches. Extracted from the small white flowers of its bushy shrub, feverfew was also used to treat inflammation caused by arthritis and for menstrual complaints.

Therapeutic Applications: headaches, migraine headaches, arthritis, menstrual pain

Scientific Updates: The anti-migraine properties of this herb have been attributed to the lactone compounds found in feverfew. Some new data questions this effect and research is continuiung. There is some speculation that the compounds in this herb manipulate serotonin, histamine and other biochemicals.

Safety: Feverfew is considered relatively safe although chewing the fresh leaves can cause swelling of the lips and tongue. Do not take feverfew while pregnant or while nursing.

Special Instructions: Taking feverfew regularly is recommended to prevent migraines but must be taken for several weeks to achieve optimal results. Store the herb in the refrigerator to preserve its active constituents.

Product Availability: Feverfew is available in dried form, and in capsules, in concentrated drops, in tinctures and in extracts. Look for supplements standardized to a 0.1 to 0.2 percent of parthenolide. One study indicated that several commercial feverfew products were missing this compound, which can also breakdown in the dried product when stored for longer periods of time. For this reason, look for products with an expiration date.

Complementary Agents: skullcap, wood betony, lavender, vervain, St. John's wort

References

Awang et al. 1991. Parthenolide content of feverfew (Tanacetum parthenium) assessed by HPLC and H-NMR spectroscopy. *Journal of Natural Products* 54(6):1516–21.

Barsby et al. 1993. Feverfew and vascular smooth muscle: extracts from fresh and dried plants show opposing pharmacological profiles, dependent upon sesquiterpene lactone content. *Planta Medica* 59(1):20–5.

Brown et al. 1997. Pharmacological activity of feverfew (Tanacetum parthenium (L.) Schultz-Bip.): assessment by inhibition of human polymorphonuclear leukocyte chemiluminescence in-vitro. *J Pharm Pharmacol* 49(5):558–61.

Heptinstall et al. 1992. Parthenolide content and bioactivity of feverfew (Tanacetum parthenium (L.) Schultz-Bip.): Estimation of commercial and authenticated feverfew products. *J. Pharm. Pharmacol* 44(5):391–95.

Garcinia *(Garcinia cambogia, or HCA)*

Overview: Indigenous to India and Thailand, garcinia has been primarily used for appetite control. It is thought to inhibit the conversion of carbohydrates into fat and to enhance thermogenesis (the conversion of calories to heat). The high hydroxycitric acid content of garcinia is believed to alter the accumulation of fatty tissue. It is thought to be one of the most effective herbal agents for the control of fat storage.

Therapeutic Actions: appetite suppressant, high cholesterol levels, endurance, energy, obesity, weight control

Scientific Updates: Recent studies suggest that garcinia can initiate fatty acid oxidation in the liver, which could prevent excess carbohydrates from turning into fat. This herb has also demonstrated the ability to inhibit adipose (fat) storage and suppress the appetite. Garcinia also encourages the build up of glycogen stores for more available energy. Laboratory studies suggest that HCA also suppresses appetite and induces weight loss. One study found that consuming one gram of the fruit containing HCA prior to each meal resulted in significant loss of weight.

Safety: At this writing, HCA is generally recognized as safe with no known toxicity, although it has not been tested in pregnant or nursing women.

Special Instructions: Dosages of HCA can vary. Taking 500 mg of HCA three times daily before each meal is customary but is below the amount used in studies. Combining HCA supplementation with a low fat diet and exercise is recommended.

Product Availability: HCA is available in capsules, powders, tablets, bars, gum and in powdered meal replacements.

Complementary Agents: gotu kola, carnitine, DHEA, chromium picolinate, coenzyme Q10

References

Greenwood et al. 1981. Effect of (-)-hydroxycitrate on development of obesity in the Zucker obese rat. *Am Phys Journal* 240:E72–78.

Heymsfield S et al. 1998. Garcinia cambogia (hydroxycitric acid) as a potential antiobesity agent. *JAMA* 280:1596–1600.

Triscari et al. 1977. Comparative effects of (-)-hydroxycitrate and (=)-allo-hydroxycitrate on acetyl CoA carboxylase and fatty acid and cholesterol synthesis in vivo. *Lipids* 12(4):357–63.

Garlic *(Allivum sativum)*

Overview: Used for millennia by Mediterranean and Asian peoples, garlic contains more than 200 chemical compounds. As a member of the lily family, it is one of the oldest cultivated plants. Sulphur substances such as allicin and ajoene are what give garlic its antibiotic properties, as well as its pungent smell. Garlic has been used for everything from treating infection, to increased sexual prowess, to parasites, to the plague.

Therapeutic Applications: arteriosclerosis, arthritis, asthma, blood poisoning, blood pressure (high or low), bronchitis, cancer, candida, circulatory insufficiency, colds, colitis, coughs, digestive disorders, ear infections, fever, flu, fungus, gas, heart disease, infections (viral and bacterial), liver ailments, lung disorders, parasites, pinworm, prostate gland disorders, respiratory congestion, yeast infections

Scientific Updates: Garlic has been the subject of intense scientific study over the last three decades (over 2,000 studies). Recent research has proven the value of garlic in treating and preventing cardiovascular disease. Controlled studies have discovered that garlic can lower cholesterol and triglyceride levels, reduce the tendency of the blood to clot, and decrease blood pressure. It has also been scientifically proven that garlic inhibits bacterial growth. One milligram of allicin, garlic's primary constituent, is estimated to equal fifteen standard units of penicillin. Dr. Erik Block discovered that garlic also protects the liver from drugs, radiation and free radical damage. Garlic can also stimulate immunity and is considered an anticancer agent.

Safety: Garlic is considered safe, but an excessive dose can cause stomach upset and gas. When using garlic directly on the skin, first coat the area with olive oil to avoid skin irritation. Do not use garlic in large amounts if you have anemia or ulcers. Garlic is a natural blood thinner; so if you are using anticoagulant drugs, check with your doctor before using garlic. There are no known contraindications to the use of garlic for pregnant or nursing women.

Special Instructions: Taking garlic with meals can help to prevent digestive upset. If you are fighting an infection, combining garlic with echinacea, goldenseal, zinc, or transfer factor is recommended.

Product Availability: Garlic is available as a fresh clove that can be chewed or juiced and in gel caps, tablets, tinctures and bulk powders. Deodorized products are available as well as enteric coated pills designed to preserve the active compounds found in garlic in the stomach. Look for products that have standardized allicin or total sulfur content.

Complementary Agents: parsley, echinacea, goldenseal, capsicum, red clover, vitamin C, bioflavonoids, olive leaf, transfer factor, proanthocyanidins

References

Avato et al. 2000. Allylsulfide constituents of garlic volatile oil as antimicrobial agents. *Phytomedicine* 7(3):239–43.

Bordia et al. 1998. Effect of garlic (Allium sativa) on blood lipids, blood sugar, fibrinogen and fibrinolytic activity in patients with coronary artery disease. *Prostaglandins Leukot Essent Fatty Acids* 58(4):257–63.

Orekhov et al. 1995. Direct anti-atherosclerosis-related effects of garlic. *Annals of Medicine* 27:63–65.

Wang et al. 1998. Protective effects of aged garlic extract against bromobenzene toxicity to precision cut rat liver slices. *Toxicology* 126(3):213–22.

Ginger *(Zingiber officinale)*

Overview: While ginger is known to most people as a pleasant tasting spice, it has been used for centuries to treat colds, nausea and joint problems. Considered a tropical plant that grows in Asia, the root or rhizome is used for both medicinal purposes and as a food spice. Ginger is most famous for its positive effect on the stomach and digestive system and for its catalyst action when combined with other herbs. It is used primarily to treat morning sickness, upset stomachs and motions sickness. In addition, it works to reduce fevers and eases cold symptoms and has recently been found to have powerful anti-inflammatory properties.

Therapeutic Applications: bronchitis, circulation, colds, colic, colitis, diarrhea, fatigue, fever, flu, headache, heart disease, indigestion, morning sickness, motion sickness, nausea, flatulence, heartburn, sore throat, stomach maladies, vomiting, joint and muscle pain, fibromyalgia

Scientific Updates: Ginger has exhibited some impressive cardio-tonic effects (lowering cholesterol) and has also shown to be valuable for alleviating stress and invigorating the body. Numerous scientific studies have been conducted on ginger. Recent findings published in *The Lancet* report the effectiveness of ginger in treating motion sickness and nausea over standard drug therapies. Researchers have also found two natural antibiotic agents in ginger. Ginger has also been described as an effective anti-inflammatory agent that works as well as non-steroidal anti-inflammatory drugs with none of their side effects. A recent study on over 100 test subjects found that ginger was as effective as metoclopramide for preventing nausea. Ginger works directly on the stomach in preventing motion sickenss, rather than going through the nervous system like Dramamine. Ginger also stimulates circulation and inhibits the formation of blood clots.

Safety: Ginger has been taken for centuries with no known toxicity or side effects. It is commonly taken by pregnant women to control morning sickness. There have not been, however, any studies on its effect on pregnant or nursing women. Taking a large dose on an empty stomach can create a slight burning sensation.

Special Instructions: Ginger is a very versatile herb. Ginger teas sweetened with honey can soothe an upset stomach. Cooking with fresh ginger helps to prevent heartburn and taking ginger capsules before you get in a boat or car can also prevent the onset of motion sickness.

Product Availability: You can buy ginger as a fresh root, in powder form, or as tablets, capsules, tinctures, essential oils, extracts, teas and syrups. Candied ginger or ginger ale made with pure ginger may also help alleviate nausea in children. Ginger oil is recommended as a massage agent for sore muscles, compromised circulation or to alleviate congestion.

Complementary Agents: capsicum, licorice, papaya, digestive enzymes, parsley, peppermint, garlic, fennel, catnip, bilberry, dandelion, ginseng, bee pollen, bee propolis

References

Cyong, J. 1982. A pharmacological study of the antiinflammatory activity of Chinese herbs—A review. *Int J Acupuncture Electro-Ther Res.* (7):173–202.

Kikuzaki et al. 1993. Antioxidant effects of some ginger constituents. *Journal of Food Science* 58:1407.

Phillips et al. 1993. Zingiber officinale (ginger): An antiemetic for day case surgery. *Anaesthesia* 48:715–17.

Qian et al. 1992. Pharmacologic studies of antimotion sickness actions of ginger. *Chung Kuo Chung Hsi I Chieh Ho Tsa Chih* 12(2):95–8, 70.

Srivastava et al. 1992. Ginger (Zingiber offincinale) in rheumatic and musculoskeletal disorders. *Medical Hypotheses* 39(4):342-8.

Vutyavanich et al. 2001. Ginger for nausea and vomiting in pregnancy: randomized, double-masked, placebo-controlled trial. *Obstet Gynecol* 97(4):577–82.

Ginkgo *(Ginkgo biloba)*

Overview: The most ancient of all trees, ginkgo grows in areas of the Far East and has been a favorite of Chinese practitioners for the treatment of respiratory disorders. Today, ginkgo is the subject of widespread scientific inquiry for its ability to increase oxygenation to brain cells as well as other body areas (especially the inner ear). It is widely used to improve mood and stimulate better brain function, and its strong antioxidant action may actually slow down the effects of aging. For this reason, it may help to prevent hearing loss, Alzheimer's disease, stroke, and depression. In addition, it may also be beneficial for varicose veins, macular degeneration, impotence and other disorders related to poor circulation.

Therapeutic Applications: Alzheimer's disease, asthma, depression, attention deficit disorder, anxiety attacks, stress, blood clots, circulatory insufficiency, dementia, kidney disease, memory loss, respiratory disease, senility, stroke, tinnitus, vascular disease, impotence, macular degeneration, varicose veins

Scientific Updates: Numerous studies have found that ginkgo can protect the neuronal membranes in the brain and help prevent the decrease in cerebral reception that occurs with aging. In an open trial involving 112 geriatric patents who suffered from inadequate cerebral blood flow, 120 mg of ginkgo extract caused a significant regression of pre-existing symptoms. A recent study also found that ginkgo helped to decrease the effects of brain hemorrhaging. A multicenter study published in the *Journal of the American Medical Association*, reported that ginkgo extract supplementation did offer benefits for the treatment of Alzheimer's disease. The brain-protective effect of ginkgo was documented in another study in which ginkgo protected brain cells from oxygen deprivation. Ginkgo can also reduce stress and anxiety and elevate mood by possibly acting like an MAO inhibitor.

Safety: Considered nontoxic and virtually without side effects, ginkgo can be safely used with other supplements. In rare cases, some gastric upset or incidence of headache or skin rash has occurred (probably indicating an allergic reaction). If you take more than 300 mg, you may experience a mild headache, dizziness or stomach upset. People taking daily aspirin to thin the blood or prescription anticoagulants such as warfarin (Coumadin) should avoid ginkgo. It appears to be safe for pregnant or nursing women although there are no studies to confirm this claim.

Special Instructions: Look for standardized capsules or other products that contain 24 percent of flavoglycosides and 6 percent terpene lactones and use as directed. Be aware that ginkgo is much more effective if taken prior to or in the very early stages of Alzheimer's disease.

Product Availability: Ginkgo is available in tablets, liquids, softgels and powdered forms. It is often added to brain, mood and memory formulas.

Complementary Agents: ginseng, gotu kola, sage, vinpocetine, bee pollen, capsicum, suma, St. John's wort, garlic, vitamin B-complex, SAMe, folic acid, magnesium, choline, DHEA

References

Kanowski et al. 1997. Proof of efficacy of the Ginkgo biloba special extract EGb 761 in outpatients suffering from mild to moderate primary degenerative dementia of the Alzheimer's type or multi-infarct dementia. *Phytomedicine* (4)1:3–13.

LeBars et al. 1997. A placebo-controlled, double-blind, randomized trial of an extract of Ginkgo biloba for dementia. *JAMA* 278:1327–32.

Smith et al. 1996. The neuroprotective properties of the Ginkgo biloba leaf: a review of the possible relationship to platelet-activating factor (PAF). *Journal of Ethnopharmacology* 50(3):131–39.

Sun et al. 2000. Effects of Ginkgo biloba extract on somatosensory evoked potential, nitric oxide levels in serum and brain tissue in rats with cerebral vasospasm after sub-arachnoid hemorrhage. *Clin Hemorheol Microcirculation* 23(2–4):139–44.

White et al. 1996. Extracts of Ginkgo biloba leaves inhibit monoamine oxidase. *Life Sciences* 58:1315–21.

Ginseng, Panax (Eleutherococcus senticosus)

Overview: Used for generations by the Chinese, Panax ginseng was traditionally taken for increasing life span and wisdom. Also known as Chinese or Korean ginseng, Panax ginseng is related to American ginseng *(Panax quinquefolium)*. Considered one of the best tonic, adaptogenic herbs, ginseng has captured the interest of the scientific community. It has been found to lower cholesterol, boost cardiovascular function, prevent blood clots, increase stamina and protect cells from radiation. It is commonly used to strengthen the sexual system, improve athletic performance and boost memory and brain function. New studies have found that it helps to regulate blood pressure, supports the adrenal glands and stabilizes blood sugar. It also has immune boosting effects.

Therapeutic Applications: allergies, aging, drug withdrawal, depression, diabetes, colds, hypertension, radiation protection, impotence, lung disorders, prostate gland disease, compromised immunity, sexual dysfunction, geriatric conditions, chronic fatigue syndrome

Scientific Updates: A study published in *The American Journal of Chinese Medicine* reports that ginseng can moderate the effects of a high-cholesterol diet in both rats and humans. Clinical testing has found that ginseng can prevent cellular damage from radiation exposure. Ginseng can also increase sperm count, lower blood sugar and help to treat alcoholism. Numerous European studies showed that athletes who took ginseng had enhanced oxygen uptake. Two other recent studies found that ginseng had a cancer preventive effect. It has also shown some promise for erectile dysfunction and chronic fatigue syndrome. Siberian ginseng may offer benefits for allergic reactions.

Safety: Generally recognized as safe, ginseng is considered nontoxic if used in reasonable amounts. Some people may have trouble sleeping or feel overstimulated while taking this herb, and some people have also reported breast tenderness and changes in the menstrual cycle. People taking high blood pressure or heart medications should not take ginseng and it is not for children or pregnant or nursing women. Note: A study published in the *Journal of the American Medical Association* in 1979 erroneously reported that ginseng causes high blood pressure and irritability. The study was subsequently discredited.

Special Instructions: Herbal practitioners typcially recommend taking ginseng for three to four weeks at a time and then taking a week off. It should not be taken for longer than three months without a break.

Product Availability: Ginseng can be purchased in extracts of whole root, teas, and capsules. You should look for standardized extracts because potency can vary. Older ginseng roots are more medicinally powerful than younger ones. Purchase concentrated products that have standardized ginsenoside contents.

Complementary Agents: gotu kola, ginkgo, fo-ti, St. John's wort, bee pollen, saw palmetto, wild yam, DHEA, vitamin B-complex, antioxidant array

References

Choi et al. 1995. Clinical efficacy of Korean red ginseng for erectile dysfunction. *Int J Impot Res* 7(3):181–6.

Jeong et al. 2001. Inhibitory effects of mast cell-mediated allergic reactions by cell cultured Siberian ginseng. *Immunopharmacol Immunotoxicol* 23(1):107–17.

Rosenfeld et al. 1984. Evaluation of the efficacy of a standardized ginseng extract in patients with psychophysical asthenia and neurological disorders. *La Semana Medica* 173:148–54.

Xiaoguang et al. 1998. Cancer chemopreventive and therapeutic activities of red ginseng. *J Ethnopharmacol* 60(1):71–8.

Yun et al. 1995. Preventive effect of ginseng intake against various human cancers: A case-control study on 1,987 pairs. *Cancer Epidemiology, Biomarkers & Prevention* 4:401–08.

Glucomannan *(Amorphophallus konjak)*

Overview: Glucomannan is a unique herb that comes from the root of the konjac plant and provides dietary fiber with no calories. It promotes bowel elimination, absorbs intestinal toxins and can help normalize blood sugar. In addition, when taken before meals, this herb can help to produce a feeling of fullness, thereby suppressing the appetite. It can expand to about fifty times its original volume when combined with water, so it is a good diet aid and source of fiber.

Therapeutic Applications: atherosclerosis, high cholesterol, constipation, sluggish colon, hypertension, diabetes, blood sugar disorders, obesity

Scientific Updates: Glucomannan is currently being used in weight reduction formulas to suppress carbohydrate cravings. When combined with lecithin, it is thought to help prevent cardiovascular disease. New studies also point to its value for insulin control, cholesterol reduction and some cases of childhood constipation. It may also help to inhibit the absorption of fat in the stomach.

Safety: Glucomanna is considered nontoxic, but anyone suffering from any blood-sugar-related disease should check with their physician before using it.

Special Instructions: Take two to three capsules with a full glass of water fifteen to twenty minutes prior to meals.

Product Availability: Glucomannan is commonly taken in capsules, although it can be purchased in loose dried form. It is frequently added to meal replacement or weight loss products.

Complementary Agents: lecithin, chromium, garcinia, garlic, hawthorn, essential fatty acids, carnatine, fiber sources (psyllium, guar gum, etc.)

References

Gallaher et al. 2000. Cholesterol reduction by glucomannan and chitosan is mediated by changes in cholesterol absorption and bile acid and fat excretion in rats. *Journal of Nutrition* 130(11):2753–9.

Staiano et al. 2000. Effect of the dietary fiber glucomannan on chronic constipation in neurologically impaired children. *J Pediatr* 136(1):41–5.

Vuksan et al. 2000. Beneficial effects of viscous dietary fiber from Konjac-mannan in subjects with the insulin resistance syndrome: results of a controlled metabolic trial. *Diabetes Care* 23(1):9–14.

Goldenseal *(Hydrastis canadensis)*

Overview: Used by Native Americans for generations, goldenseal root is a favorite among herbalists for its natural anti-inflammatory effect and antibiotic-like actions. The bitter nature of this herb has made it an effective remedy for digestive disorders. It is also used as a bitter tonic for gastric ulcers. Strained infusions of goldenseal have traditionally been used as a soothing eye wash. Its growing popularity has caused a number of states to place it on an endangered plant list. Goldenseal can be used both internally and externally. Its berberine content fights disease microorgansims and parasites; and topically, it acts as an antiseptic for wounds, canker sores, etc.

Therapeutic Applications: Internal: diarrhea, eczema, eye inflammations, flatulence, gallbladder disease, gastritis, giardia, hemorrhoids, impetigo, indigestion, infections (viral and bacterial), liver disease, excessive menstrual flow, parasites, urinary tract infections, mouth sores, rhinitis, ringworm, ulcers, vaginitis, yeast infections External: wounds, abrasions, bug bites, stings, cuts, rashes, boils, sores

Scientific Updates: Laboratory tests have proven goldenseal's ability to protect against gram-positive and gram-negative bacteria, including tuberculosis bacteria. It helps to reduce vaginal and uterine inflammation, and stuides have found that berberine-containing herbs (such as goldenseal) can be more effective in treating gastrointestinal infections than standard antibiotics. Studies have recently investigated how berberine inhibits cancer cells and reduces inflammation. In addition, berberine has been found to be more effective in treating malaria-related parasites than tetracycline.

Safety: Prolonged or excessive use of goldenseal may kill bacterial flora and raise white blood count. Taking unusually high amounts of goldenseal can lower heartbeat and adversely effect the central nervous system. Pregnant or nursing women should not use this herb as its berberine content can stimulate uterine contractions. Continual use can lower vitamin B absorption. Goldenseal is not recommended for anyone with low blood sugar or hypertension.

Special Instructions: If taking goldenseal for an infection, you may want to combine it with echinacea, garlic and elderberry for optimal results. Goldenseal is also commonly mixed with myrrh and dandelion in topical ointments.

Product Availability: The most common forms of goldenseal are liquid extracts and capsules. Look for products with standardized berberine content.

Complementary Agents: barberry, Oregon grape, echinacea, garlic, capsicum, myrrh, ginger, eyebright, juniper, dandelion, chamomile, black cohosh, comfrey, cascara sagrada, gentian, dong quai, vitamin C, bioflavonoids, transfer factor, vitamin A, digestive enzymes, grape seed or pine bark proanthocyanidins

References

Berberine. 2000. *Altern Med Rev* 5(2):175–7.

Rehman et al. 1999. Increased production of antigen-specific immunoglobulins G and M following in vivo treatment with the medicinal plants Echinacea angustifolia and Hydrastis canadensis. *Immunol Lett.* 1:68(2–3):391–5.

Sheng et al. 1997. Treatment of chloroquine-resistant malaria using pyrimethamine in combination with berberine, tetracycline or cotrimoxazole. *East Afr Med J* 74(5):283–4.

Wu et al. 1998. Inhibitory effects of berberine on voltage- and calcium-activated potassium currents in human myeloma cells. *Life Sci* 62(25):2283–94.

Gotu Kola (Centella asiatica)

Overview: Grown in Java and Ceylon, gotu kola is one of the most popular Ayurvedic (Indian) herbs. It is utilized as a nerve tonic, a remedy for epilepsy and as a brain normalizer in conditions such as memory loss and schizophrenia. It was also suggested for depression, fatigue and to boost circulation. Recently, scientists have discovered its ability to treat inflammation and fever. Gotu kola is often referred to as centella and should not be confused with a caffeine-containing herb called kola nut. Externally, gotu kola is also beneficial for wounds, burns and psoriasis.

Therapeutic Applications: age-related disorders, arteriosclerosis, circulatory problems, epilepsy, high blood pressure, depression, fatigue, hypoglycemia, learning disorders, memory loss, menopause, nervous conditions, PMS, psoriasis, schizophrenia, senility, ulcerations, wounds

Scientific Updates: Gotu kola contains triterpenoid compounds, which may account for its therapeutic properties. Studies have indicated that gotu kola works as a tonic for fatigue without the side effects of caffeine. It also stimulates and builds the nervous system, thus counteracting the effects of stress. Europeans and Asians use this herb for psoriasis and vaginitis. In India, gotu kola has enjoyed widespread use as a brain food, with a therapeutic focus on improving memory and promoting longevity. Other studies have shown that gotu kola causes a gradual increase in blood sugar levels, which may benefit people with hypoglycemia who also battle behavioral symptoms related to insulin and blood sugar.

Safety: Gotu kola is considered generally safe. Recent studies have found the herb to be nontoxic even at relatively high dosages. At high doses, some people have experienced headaches, insomnia or an overactive mind. Interestingly, at high doses it can also have a sedative effect. Gotu kola should not be used by pregnant or nursing women.

Special Instructions: Some herbalists recommend that after six weeks on this herb, it's wise to take a two-week break.

Product Availability: Gotu kola is commonly found in combination products designed to boost mood and energy. It is available as a single supplement in powders, capsules and liquid extracts. Look for supplements with standardized levels of triterpenes, (asiaticoside and asiatic acid) at 2 to 4 percent.

Complementary Agents: ginseng, ginkgo, capsicum, licorice, St. John's wort, fo-ti, vitamin C, bioflavonoids, SAMe, vitamin E, vitamin D, zinc, bee pollen and bee propolis

References

Bradwejn et al. 2000. A double-blind, placebo-controlled study on the effects of Gotu Kola (Centella asiatica) on acoustic startle response in healthy subjects. *J Clin Psychopharmacol* 20(6):680–4.

Cauffield, J. 1999. Dietary supplements used in the treatment of depression, anxiety, and sleep disorders. *Lippincotts Prim Care Pract* 3(3):290–304.

Cesarone et al. 1994. The microcirculatory activity of Centella asiatica in venous insufficiency. A double-blind study. *Minerva Cardioangiol* 42(6):299–304.

Suguna et al. 1996. Effects of Centella asiatica extract on dermal wound healing in rats. *Indian J Exp Biol* 34(12):1208–11.

Green Tea *(Camellia sinensis)*

Overview: Green tea is made from the young leaves of the *Camellia sinensis* bush, which is very popular in Asia. Black tea is made from the same plant but is a processed form and does not have the same nutrient profile as green tea. Used for millennia by practitioners for respiratory ailments and for mental rejuvenation, western scientists have validated its remarkable antioxidant actions due to compounds called catechins. It not only offers cancer protection, but also can inhibit the formation of blood clots, lower cholesterol levels, stabilize blood sugar and boost the burning of fat.

Therapeutic Applications: weight loss, cholesterol control, cancer prevention, cancer treatment, augmentative for chemotherapy

Scientific Updates: New studies have found that the more green tea one consumes, the better chance for recovery from certain types of breast cancer. Green tea has shown that it can actually inhibit the growth of tumors that affect the breast, colon and lung. In addition, topical applications of green tea can protect the skin against sun-induced damage. In one study, green tea was tested in cancerous mice who were also given a chemotherapy drug. The results suggest that green tea may better a patient's overall health during chemotherapy treatments.

Safety: Green tea contains caffeine in small amounts (approximately 20 to 30 mg per cup). The caffeine content of most supplementary capsules is usually half this. If you have any adverse effects to caffeine, you should not use green tea. People with nervous conditions, insomnia, etc., are generally advised to avoid caffeine.

Special Instructions: Make sure the supplement you purchase does not have added caffeine or you may experience nervousness or insomnia.

Product Availability: Green tea is most often taken in tea form made with the loose herb or with tea bag products. It can also be purchased as encapsulated extracts. Look for supplements that are standardized to a 25 percent or higher content of polyphenols. Green tea extracts are also added to a number of cosmetics including sun blocks, hair products and hand lotions.

Complementary Agents: grapeseed or pinebark extracts, beta-carotene, vitamin C with bioflavonoids, vitamin E, garlic

References

Dulloo et al. 1996. Tealine and thermogenesis: Interaction between polyphenols, caffeine and sympathetic activity. *International Journal of Obesity* 20(S4):71.

Katiyar et al. 1999. Polyphenolic antioxidant (-)-epigallocatechin-3-gallate from green tea reduces UVB-induced inflammatory responses and infiltration of leukocytes in human skin. *Photochem Photobiol* 69(2):148–53.

Kuroda et al. 1999. Antimutagenic and anticarcinogenic activity of tea polyphenols. *Mutat Res* 436(1):69–97.

Nakachi et al. 1998. Influence of drinking green tea on breast cancer malignancy among Japanese patients. *Jpn J Cancer Res* 89(3):254–61.

Guarana (Paullinia cupana)

Overview: Also known as Brazilian cocoa, guarana contains a compound virtually identical to caffeine and has been used as an energy drink and natural stimulant. Guarana contains chemical compounds called xanthines, which include caffeine, theobromine and theophylline. Herbal practitioners traditionally used guarana for diarrhea, arthritis and to suppress appetite. This herb directly stimulates the central nervous system and can also have a diuretic effect.

Therapeutic Applications: appetite suppressant, aphrodisiac, diarrhea, fatigue, gastrointestinal disorders, headaches, migraines, neuralgia, PMS, athletic endurance, obesity

Scientific Updates: Guarana is used for its stimulating properties and for its diuretic action. It is also considered an antidiarrheic and antifatigue agent. Its potential for treating migraine headaches is under current investigation. It can harm a developing fetus, increase metabolic rate and like caffeine, may negatively impact blood vessels.

Safety: Pregnant women and nursing mothers should not use guarana. Overuse can cause a strain on the urinary tract, urinary frequency, hyperactivity, heart palpitations or insomnia. Combining guarana with herbs like ephedra can create anxiety and heart arrythmias. People with high blood pressure, heart disease or anxiety disorders should not use this herb. As is the case with caffeine, long-term use may cause compromised fertility, heart problems and even cancer. Be aware that using guarana with Chinese ephedra improperly can cause serious health concerns.

Special Instructions: Guarana can be taken as a single supplement but is usually included in weight loss formulas or energy combinations. A cup of guarana tea can be made by placing 1 to 2 grams of the crushed seed in 1 cup of water and boiling for ten minutes. Three cups a day are customary. You should not consume over 200 mg of guarana daily, and you should not take it for long periods of time.

Product Availability: Guarana is available as crushed seeds or resin, in capsules, extracts, tinctures or teas. Look for products with a standardized guaranine content.

Complementary Agents: yerba maté, ginseng, gotu kola, garcinia, kola nut, chickweed

References:

Duke, J.A. 1985. *CRC Handbook of Medicinal Herbs* Boca Raton, FL: CRC Press. p.349.

Galduroz et al. 1996. The effects of long-term administration of guarana on the cognition of normal, elderly volunteers. *Rev Paul Med* 114:1073–8.

Miura et al. 1998. Effect of guarana on exercise in normal and epinephrine-induced glycogenolytic mice. *Biol Pharm Bull* 21(6):646–8.

Ooms et al. 2001. Suspected caffeine and ephedrine toxicosis resulting from ingestion of an herbal supplement containing guarana and ma huang in dogs: 47 cases (1997-1999). *J Am Vet Med Assoc* 15:218(2):225–9.

Gymnema *(Gymnema sylvestre)*

Overview: Gymnema leaves come from trees native to Africa and India that belong to the milkweed family. They have the remarkable ability to block out certain taste sensations, especially sweetness. Gymnema is an extremely popular herb in Japan and is included in diabetic, hypoglycemic and weight-loss formulas. In some ancient languages, its name signifies "destroyer of sugar."

Therapeutic Applications: diabetes, fatigue, hypoglycemia, insulin resistance obesity, sugar cravings, high cholesterol

Scientific Updates: Modern research has found that gymnemic acid, the active ingredient of the herb, blocks sugar absorption in the body. A clinical study published in 1986 suggests that extract of gymnema can significantly enhance liver and pancreatic function. Both human and animal studies confirm that gymnema effects blood sugar levels especially in diabetics. It has been suggested that it might be of value even as a treatment for Type I diabetes. It not only lowers blood glucose levels, but cholesterol and blood fat levels as well.

Safety: Diabetics should check with their physician before using this herb and never discontinue insulin or other treatments in exchange for an herbal therapy without the consent and supervision of their doctor. If you take gymnema, you may have to lower the dosage of your other antidiabetic drugs. It is also thought that fenfluramine and possibly other antidepressant drugs that raise serotonin levels, salicylates (including aspirin) and tetracyclines may potentiate the action of gymnema. On the contrary, its therapeutic properties may be decreased by thyroid medications, oral contraceptives, phenothiazines and epinephrine.

Special Instructions: If you already have problems with hypoglycemia, you may want to experiment with this herb. Be aware that taking gymnema is no license to overeat sugar or starchy foods, especially if you have a blood sugar disorder.

Product Availability: Gymnema is commonly taken in capsule form.

Complementary Agents: fenugreek, goldenseal, milk thistle, ginger, bilberry, blueberry, dandelion, vitamin C, vitamin A, B-complex, bioflavonoids, proanthocyanidins, chromium, bee pollen, bee propolis

References

Persaud et al. 1999. Gymnema sylvestre stimulates insulin release in vitro by increased membrane permeability. *J Endocrinol* 163(2):207–12.

Preuss et al. 1998. Comparative effects of chromium, vanadium and gymnema sylvestre on sugar-induced blood pressure elevations in SHR. *J Am Coll Nutr* 17(2):116–23.

Sugihara et al. 2000. Antihyperglycemic effects of gymnemic acid IV, a compound derived from Gymnema sylvestre leaves in streptozotocin-diabetic mice. *J Asian Nat Prod Res* 2(4):321–7.

Wang et al. 1998. Inhibitory effect of gymnemic acid on intestinal absorption of oleic acid in rats. *Can J Physiol Pharmacol* 76(10–11):1017–23.

Hawthorn Berry *(Crataegus oxyacantha)*

Overview: Hawthorn berry has been utilized as a medicinal remedy since the time of the ancient Greeks. Known as a botanical heart tonic, hawthorn berry was traditionally used to treat high and low blood pressure, irregular heartbeat, heart pain and atherosclerosis. Native Americans looked to the berry for its therapeutic effect on rheumatism and digestive difficulties. Hawthorn is considered one of the best botanical heart tonics available and is widely used by doctors in European countries like Germany. It also has significant antioxidant and anti-inflammatory properties and strengthens collagen.

Therapeutic Applications: angina, irregular heartbeat, blood pressure disorders, congestive heart failure, hypertension, coronary artery disease, high cholesterol, nervous disorders, insomnia, Reynaud's syndrome, sore throat, joint diseases, collagen-related diseases (weakness)

Scientific Updates: The cardio-tonic properties of hawthorn are well documented. The flavonoid content of the berry has been clinically shown to dilate peripheral and coronary blood vessels, which helps alleviate hypertension and angina. Experimental studies have found that hawthorn works in three important ways: it eases blood flow, lowers blood pressure and strengthens heart muscle. One of the most desirable benefits of hawthorn is that its heart-protective role may actually increase when the herb is used for a prolonged period of time. In addition, hawthorn has the ability to lower serum cholesterol levels and to prevent cholesterol deposits from accumulating in arteries. It is also an extremely valuable therapeutic agent for the early stages of congestive heart failure and arrhythmia. Scientists have reported that its powerful antioxidant properties are very beneficial to overall circulatory health. A German study found that hawthorn gently increases the strength of the heart, normalizes rhythm, and benefits circulation within the heart itself by dilating the coronary arteries.

Safety: No known toxicity has been found in hawthorn. It may potentiate the action of digitalis and should only be mixed with pharmaceutical drugs when approved by a physician. The effects of hawthorn can be cumulative. Its effect on pregnant or nursing women is unknown.

Special Instructions: Take hawthorn capsules or tincture with food. Hawthorn is not a short-term remedy. It is a slow-acting cardio tonic; its value is best utilized through long-term use.

Product Availability: Hawthorn leaf is available in liquid and dry extracts for oral intake. The dried berries can also used to make an infusion with boiling water.

Complementary Agents: capsicum, grapeseed or pinebark extract, garlic, passionflower, valerian, peppermint, ginkgo, vitamin C, vitamin A, vitamin E, vitamin B-complex, calcium/magnesium, potassium, selenium, coenzyme Q10, marine lipids or essential fatty acids

References

Holubarsch et al. 2000. Survival and prognosis: investigation of Crataegus extract WS 1442 in congestive heart failure (SPICE)—rationale, study design and study protocol. *Eur J Heart Fail* 2(4):431–7.

Rothfuss et al. 2001. Effect of long-term application of Crataegus oxyacantha on ischemia and reperfusion induced arrhythmias in rats. *Arzneimittelforschung* 51(1):24–8.

Schwinger et al. 2000. Crataegus special extract WS 1442 increases force of contraction in human myocardium cAMP-independently. *J Cardiovasc Pharmacol* 5(5):700–7.

Ho-Shou-Wu *(Polygonum multiflorum)*

Overview: Traditionally used by the Chinese to promote longevity, this herb is rich in flavonoids and is primarily used to restore vigor, strengthen the cardiovascular system, enhance the endocrine system and tone the liver and kidneys. It is also good for chronic fatigue or degenerative conditions.

Therapeutic Applications: aging, cardiovascular conditions, chronic fatigue, circulatory insufficiency, debilitating conditions, glandular disorders, impotency, infertility

Scientific Updates: Research on this herb is limited; however, it has shown promise for amnesia and for oxygenating heart muscle. It has also demonstrated impressive antioxidant actions in scientific studies. Its long history of use by the Chinese in restorative herbal formulas attests to its tonic action.

Safety: This herb is presumed to be safe; however, there are no studies establishing its safety for pregnant or nursing mothers or its potential for drug interactions. There is documented evidence that a batch of ho-shou-wu caused an outbreak of hepatitis. Unprocessed ho-shou-wu may cause a mild diarrhea. Make sure to get this herb from reliable sources.

Special Instructions: The usual dose of ho-shou-wu is greater than for most herbs; therefore, capsules containing small amounts of this herb are not recommended. Use as directed.

Product Availability: You can purchase this herb in tablet, capsule or tincture form.

Complementary Agents: hawthorn, garlic, coenzyme Q10, marine lipids, essential fatty acids, capsicum, vitamin E

References

Chen et al. 1999. 2,2-Diphenyl-1-picrylhydrazyl radical-scavenging active components from Polygonum multiflorum thunb. J *Agric Food Chem* 47(6):2226–8.

Hsieh et al. 2000. The ameliorating effects of the cognitive-enhancing Chinese herbs on scopolamine-induced amnesia in rats. *Phytother Res* 14(5):375–7.

Park et al. 2001. Acute hepatitis induced by Shou-Wu-Pian, a herbal product derived from Polygonum multiflorum. *J Gastroenterol Hepatol* 16(1):115–7.

Yim et al. 2000. Myocardial protection against ischaemia-reperfusion injury by a Polygonum multiflorum extract supplemented 'Dang-Gui decoction for enriching blood', a compound formulation, ex vivo. *Phytother Res* 14(3):195–9.

Hops *(Humulus lupulus)*

Overview: Hops is best known for its use in beer brewing. It is also an extremely useful nervine herb, which has traditionally been used to calm the central nervous system and safely induce sleep. During the reign of King George, it was used to fill pillows to help promote relaxation during illness. Native Americans utilized hops for an overly acidic stomach and indigestion.

Therapeutic Applications: insomnia, headaches, hyperactivity, anxiety, fever, nervousness, pain, stress, stomach spasms, inflammation, and colon disorders, lack of appetite, anorexia

Scientific Updates: Recent in-depth clinical studies reveal that hops relaxes smooth muscle and naturally sedates the nervous system. Lupulone and humulone, the active ingredients of hops, are responsible for its sedative properties. Its high flavonoid content gives hops its anti-inflammatory action and makes it a good antioxidant agent. Scientists have also found that xanthohumol, a flavonoid in the female inflorescences (cones) of hops, may have potential cancer-chemopreventive properties. Another study found that flavonoids found in hops actually inhibited the activity of a known carcinogen.

Safety: Hops has no known toxicity. It is not recommended for anyone who is suffering from clinical depression. Large quantities can have an aphrodisiac effect. There are no known contraindications or interactions of hops with other medications. If you are prone to pollen allergies, you may develop a rash from touching the dried herb. Hops should not be combined with alcoholic beverages or other depressants. Some herbalists recommend that pregnant women or those who have estrogen-dependent breast cancer should avoid using hops because it may contain estrogen-like chemicals. Avoid hops while nursing.

Special Instructions: Hops tea can be made by pouring 1 cup boiling water over 2 teaspoons of the dried herb. Steep for fifteen minutes before drinking. Tinctures are commonly taken in 1 to 2 ml two or three times per day. Capsule products are taken at a dose of 500 to 1,000 mg two times daily.

Product Availability: Hops is available as a bath additive, concentrated drops, a decoction, powder, dried herb, an extract, a fruit (fresh dried), and an infusion. Because hops has only mild sedating actions, it is most commonly used in herbal combinations containing valerian, kava, skullcap or passionflower for insomnia or agitation.

Complementary Agents: valerian root, skullcap, kava, chamomile, mullein, marshmallow, wood betony, passionflower, vitamin E, B-complex, folic acid, niacin, vitamin C, inositol, calcium/magnesium, and melatonin

References

Foster, S. 1996. *Herbs for Your Health*. Loveland, CO: Interweave Press. p. 56–7.

Milligan et al. 2000. The endocrine activities of 8-prenylnaringenin and related hop (Humulus lupulus L.) flavonoids. *J Clin Endocrinol Metab* 85(12):4912–5.

Vonderheid-Guth et al. 2000. Pharmacodynamic effects of valerian and hops extract combination (Ze 91019) on the quantitative-topographical EEG in healthy volunteers. *Eur J Med Res* 19:5(4):139–44.

Horehound *(Marrubium vulgare)*

Overview: Since ancient Roman times, horehound has been a valuable cough and cold remedy. Egyptians called it the Seed of Horus, using it as an antidote for poisons. It was also one of the bitter herbs eaten at the feast of the Passover. Horehound has been used for a wide variety of ailments including whooping cough, asthma, diarrhea, jaundice, painful menstruation and constipation.

Therapeutic Applications: bronchitis, sore throat, whooping cough, asthma, common cold, jaundice, amenorrhea, and respiratory infection

Scientific Updates: Researchers have shown that horehound exhibits antispasmodic and antinociceptive activity. They believe it has potential as a treatment for muscle spasm and general convulsions.

Safety: Studies have shown that up to five cups of horehound tea in one day is a safe dosage. Very large doses may cause abnormal heart rhythms, so you should avoid the herb if you have pre-existing heart conditions.

Special Instructions: Horehound in lozenge form is recommended for hacking coughs accompanied by sore throats. Hot tea preparations are also good for congestion and combining horehound with ginger is very good for colds and flu.

Product Availability: Horehound is available fresh, dried, powdered or as a pressed juice, liquid extract or tea.

Complementary Agents: ginger, coltsfoot, lobelia, elecampane, wild cherry bark, mullein, eucalyptus

References

Bartarelli, M. 1966. Marrubium vulgare and its pharmaceutical uses. *Boll Chim Farm* 105(11):787–98.

De Jesus et al. 2000. Analysis of the antinociceptive properties of marrubiin isolated from Marrubium vulgare. *Phytomedicine* 7(2):111–5.

Horse Chestnut *(Aesculus hippocastanum)*

Overview: For centuries eastern cultures have used horse chestnut to treat a wide range of ailments—from colds to whooping cough to rheumatism. This herb is noted for its ability to strengthen the blood vessels of the circulatory system. Horse chestnut is also a popular remedy for inflammation and swelling in varicose veins and hemorrhoids.

Therapeutic Applications: venous insufficiency, varicose veins, hemorrhoids, lower back pain, premenstrual syndrome, painful injuries, sprains, bruises and spinal problems.

Scientific Updates: Research has documented that horse chestnut seed extracts often alleviate the signs of chronic venous insufficiency. A compound called aescin is thought to be responsible. Another recent study found marked difference in the anti-inflammatory effect of horse chestnut over placebo. Other studies have found that it is an effective treatment for varicose veins.

Safety: High doses of horse chestnut can be dangerous, causing symptoms such as diarrhea, severe thirst, visual disturbances, loss of consciousness and enlarged pupils. If you suspect an overdose, get medical attention immediately. Do not crush or eat unprocessed horse chestnuts.

Special Instructions: Follow the dosage instructions on product packaging carefully. Internal doses that are too large can cause side effects. Using this herb both internally and in external applications is recommended for optimal results. For hemorrhoids, use ointments or tinctures. Lotions can be applied directly to varicose veins.

Product Availability: Internal: capsule, extract, injection, solution, pill External: gel, lotion, ointment, powder. Look for products with standardized 18 to 27 percent aescin content.

Complementary Agents: hawthorn, linden, ginkgo, yarrow

References
Bielanski et al. 1999. Horse-chestnut seed extract for chronic venous insufficiency. *J Fam Pract* 48(3):171–2.

Brunner et al. 2001. Responsiveness of human varicose saphenous veins to vasoactive agents. *Br J Clin Pharmacol* 51(3):219–24.

Loew et al. 2000. Measurement of the bioavailability of aescin-containing extracts. *Methods Find Exp Clin Pharmacol* 22(7):537–42.

Horsetail *(Equisetum arvense)*

Overview: This herb, also known as shavegrass, was used for centuries to treat internal and external injuries. Horsetail has a high silica content and helps to facilitate the use of calcium in the body. It is particularly good for boosting circulation, reducing hemorrhage, promoting the healing of wounds and broken bones, and for treating kidney and urinary tract diseases. Horsetail is considered a natural diuretic and astringent.

Therapeutic Applications: arthritis, bladder ailments, bedwetting, conjunctivitis, bone injuries, osteoarthritis, osteoporosis, glandular disorders, hair loss, kidney stones, nervous tension, tumors, urinary problems, prostatitis, brittle nails, water retention

Scientific Updates: Researchers have found that horsetail contains antibiotic and hemolytic (blood clotting) properties. Its rich array of minerals makes it ideal for the healing of injured tissue and bone. It is rich in silica, which helps strengthen connective tissue and may help with arthritis. It is especially effective in poultice form. In a recent study, scientists found that horsetail may inhibit methane production in the human digestive system. Studies have also noted horsetail's ability to improve cell protein processing. Its bioflavonoids have a diuretic effect.

Safety: Horsetail is generally considered safe for human consumption. High doses are not recommended because of the very small amounts of nicotine contained in the plant. It may also cause dermatitis in sensitive people. Pregnant or nursing women should not use this herb. Make sure not to mistake horsetail for *Equisetum palustre*, which is considered a poisonous substance. In addition, check that the enzyme *thiaminase* is not found in a horsetail supplement as it destroys the B-vitamin called thiamin. Supplements that have been processed at 100°C temperatures are preferable.

Special Instructions: Horsetail tea can be taken daily. Tinctures are commonly used at 2 to 6 ml daily. Be sure to drink plenty of fluids while taking horsetail. If you have a major skin disorder, fever, infectious disease, heart problems or abnormal muscle tension, consult a doctor before using horsetail as a bath additive.

Product Availability: Horsetail is available as a dried herb, an extract, and a tincture in most health food stores.

Complementary Agents: ginseng, marshmallow, plantain, alfalfa, yucca, dandelion, parsley, saw palmetto, glucosamine, chondroitin, shark cartilage, vitamin C, HCL, phosphorus, calcium/magnesium, hydrangea

References

Fabre et al. 1993. Thiaminase activity in Equisetum arvense and its extracts. *Plant Med Phytother* 26:190–97.

Graefe et al. 1999. Urinary metabolites of flavonoids and hydroxycinnamic acids in humans after application of a crude extract from Equisetum arvense. *Phytomedicine* 6(4):239–46.

Kiseleva, T.L. Related Articles

Horsetail. 1991. *Med Sestra* 50(3):56–9. Russian.

Leung, A.Y., and S. Foster. 1996. *Encyclopedia of Common Natural Ingredients Used in Foods, Drugs, and Cosmetics, 2nd ed.* New York: John Wiley & Sons. p. 306–8.

Seaborn, C. and F. Nielsen. 1993. Silicon: a nutritional beneficence for bones, brains and blood vessels. *Nutr Today* 28:13–18.

Hydrangea *(Hydrangea arborescens)*

Overview: *Hydrangea arborescens* is a woody-stemmed shrub native to eastern North America. It is often confused with other Hydrangea species *macrophylla, hortensis* and *quercifolia*. Native Americans used hydrangea as a diuretic, a cathartic, emetic, and treatment for wounds, burns, cancers, and other external ailments. Its most popular application was for the treatment of an inflamed or enlarged prostrate gland. It may also be useful for cystitis.

Therapeutic Applications: diuretic, detoxification, allergy, tonic, kidney stones and gravel in the urine, prostate disease, malaria, aluminum toxicity

Scientific Updates: Several studies suggest that compounds found in the Hydrangea family of plants have significant antimalarial properties. In addition, hydrangea extracts have demonstrated the ability to inhibit the release of histamine, which causes inflammation and allergic symptoms. In addition, certain chemicals in the hydrangea family help to protect the body from the toxic effects of aluminum.

Safety: In large doses, hydrangea can cause stomach pain, dizziness and vertigo. Take special care to avoid the flower buds; they contain hydrangin, which has been identified as a cyanide poison. Contacting the herb directly can cause dermatitis.

Special Instructions: For kidney stones, hydrangea is often combined with stone root, bearberry and gravel root. For prostate problems it combines well with horsetail and saw palmetto. Take hydrangea supplements only as directed.

Product Availability: Hydrangea is available as a liquid extract, syrup, or dried or powdered root (either loose or capsulized).

Complementary Agents: stone root, bearberry, gravel root, horsetail, saw palmetto

References

Avenel-Audran et al. 2000. Allergic contact dermatitis from hydrangea—is it so rare? *Contact Dermatitis* 43(4):189–91.

Kamei et al. 2000. Anti-malarial activity of leaf-extract of hydrangea macrophylla, a common Japanese plant. Acta Med Okayama. 54(5):227–32.

Ma, J. 2000. Role of organic acids in detoxification of aluminum in higher plants. *Plant Cell Physiol* 41(4):383–90.

Hyssop (Hyssopus officinalis)

Overview: Hyssop has been around since biblical times; it is mentioned in the bible as a cleansing agent. Hyssop is a member of the mint family and has been used for a variety of ailments from respiratory congestion to a stomach tonic. American herbalists used infusions of hyssop externally for relief of rheumatism, bruises and cuts. Hyssop contains camphor, which can be used to treat muscle spasms.

Therapeutic Applications: bronchitis, unproductive cough, asthma, rheumatism, upset stomach, common cold, anxiety, hysteria, petit mal, muscle spasms (backaches, etc.), HIV

Scientific Updates: In several studies, scientists have found that a compound isolated from hyssop exhibited strong anti-HIV-1 activity and have remarked on the compound's potential as a treatment for AIDS.

Safety: Taken in moderation, hyssop causes no known adverse reactions in humans, although one study noted that certain commercial preparations of hyssop cause convulsive reactions in laboratory rats. Hyssop may also cause allergic reactions in some people.

Special Instructions: Using hyssop in essential oil form makes an excellent massage medium for backaches and other muscle spasms.

Product Availability: Hyssop is available as dried leaf, infusion, liquid extract, oil, tea bag, tincture, compress, gargle, oil (external) and as a poultice.

Complementary Agents: horehound, coltsfoot, boneset, elder flower, peppermint

References

Burkhard et al. 1999. Plant-induced seizures: reappearance of an old problem. *J Neurol* 246(8):667–70.

Gollapudi et al. 1995. Isolation of a previously unidentified polysaccharide (MAR-10) from Hyssop officinalis that exhibits strong activity against human immunodeficiency virus type 1. *Biochem Biophys Res Commun* 5:210(1):145–51.

Indigo Wild *(Baptisia tinctoria)*

Overview: The root of the wild indigo plant contains its medicinal compounds. It grows in parts of the midwest and was traditionally used to make blue dye, treat gum and mouth diseases, sore throats and ulcers. It was even used to treat typhoid fever, a potentially fatal disease.

Therapeutic Applications: common cold/sore throat, Crohn's disease, ulcers, gingivitis, influenza

Scientific Updates: Scientists found that two substances isolated from indigo root exhibited strong antibacterial activity, especially against *Heliobacter pylori* bacteria, which can cause stomach ulcers. Another study found that it contained natural anti-inflammatory agents. The polysaccharides and proteins in wild indigo are believed to stimulate the immune system.

Safety: Indigo can produce nausea and vomiting. Long-term use of this herb or taking more than recommended dosages is not recommended. It should not be used by pregnant or nursing women or anyone who will be undergoing general anesthesia for surgery.

Special Instructions: Wild indigo is rarely taken as a single supplement and is often combined with echinacea and goldenseal. You may use a tincture in the amount of 1 to 2 ml three times per day but do not take it on an empty stomach or nausea may occur. Indigo can cause urine to become purplish in color.

Product Availability: Indigo is generally used in tincture form. Taking it as a single supplement is not recommended.

Complementary Agents: goldenseal, echinacea, cat's claw, olive leaf, garlic, transfer factor, zinc, vitamin C, vitamin A

References

Beuscher, N. and L. Kopanski. 1985. Stimulation of immunity by the contents of Baptisia tinctoria. *Planta Med* 5:381–84.

Kataoka et al. 2001. Antibacterial action of tryptanthrin and kaempferol, isolated from the indigo plant (Polygonum tinctorium Lour.), against Helicobacter pylori-infected Mongolian gerbils. *J Gastroenterol* 36(1):5–9.

Juniper *(Juniperus communis)*

Overview: Known for its aromatic blue-green berries, juniper has long been used in European circles to treat kidney disorders, urinary tract infections and prostate disease. It has blood purifying and antiseptic properties, which make it a natural for any disorders affecting the urinary system. Juniper berries have also been used to treat gout, warts and even cancer.

Therapeutic Applications: adrenal gland disorders, arthritis and rheumatism, bedwetting, bladder problems, colds, cystitis, diabetes, fungal infections, hypoglycemia, bacterial infections, kidney infections, kidney stones, pancreas deficiencies, water retention

Scientific Updates: Juniper acts directly on kidney function by stimulating urine flow and increasing the rate of glomerulus filtration (blood purification). Studies have found that after kidney disease, juniper can help restore kidney tissue and normalize blood pressure. Scientists have also found that a compound isolated from juniper leaves has a strong antifungal activity against candida and aspergillus fungi. It may also be effective against the herpes virus and may have liver-protective properties.

Safety: Long-term (over 6 weeks) or excessive use may cause kidney irritation or inhibited iron absorption. Do not use juniper if you have kidney disease. Using juniper in herbal blends helps to avoid this possibility. One study mentions the antifertility effects of juniper fruits. Do not take this herb if you are using diuretic drugs. Application of the essential oil directly to skin can cause a rash. Pregnant women should avoid juniper as it may cause uterine contractions.

Special Instructions: For juniper tea, steep 15 grams of berries in 1 cup of boiling water for twenty minutes in a covered container and drink two cups daily. One gram can be taken three times daily in capsule form, or 1 to 2 ml of tincture can be taken three times daily.

Product Availability: For internal use, Juniper is available as an infusion, liquid extract, oil, spirit, syrup and tincture. For external use, it comes in spirits, tar form or in bath salts. Juniper is often combined with other diuretic and antimicrobial herbs designed to treat the urinary tract.

Complementary Agents: cornsilk, uva ursi, cranberry, parsley, alfalfa, marshmallow, kelp, buchu, queen of the meadow, vitamin C, bioflavonoids, proanthocyanidins, B-complex, vitamin E, magnesium, potassium, copper, mineral and electrolyte supplements

References

Jones et al. 1998. Dietary juniper berry oil minimizes hepatic reperfusion injury in the rat. *Hepatology* 28(4):1042–50.

Kinyanjui et al. 2000. Potential antitermite compounds from Juniperus procera extracts. *Chemosphere* 41(7):1071–4.

Loehle et al. 1999. Diterpenes from the berries of Juniperus excelsa. *Phytochemistry* 50(7):1195–9.

Markkanen et al. 1981. Antiherpetic agent from juniper tree (Juniperus communis), its purification, identification and testing in primary human amnion cell cultures. *Drugs Exptl Clin Res* 7:691–7.

Tyler, V.E. 1994. *Herbs of Choice: The Therapeutic Use of Phytomedicinals.* Binghamton, NY: Pharmaceutical Products Press. p. 76–7.

Kava Kava *(Piper methysticum)*

Overview: A root native to the South Pacific, kava has been used for centuries as a calmative botanical. Its primary usage is to relax the central nervous system and promote sleep. Kava is a leafy tropical plant (Piper methysticum) in the pepper family, and kava is also the name given a pungent sedative beverage prepared from its roots. Native people drink kava as part of several rituals and to treat a variety of diseases such as cystitis, fatigue, headaches, stomach upset and whooping cough. Applied topically, kava is used to treat insect bites and stings and skin inflammations. Kava appears to offer a safe and effective alternative to prescription drugs for insomnia and anxiety without adversely affecting mental function.

Therapeutic Actions: insomnia, nervousness, stress, headaches, anxiety

Scientific Updates: Research has found that kava has mild psychoactive properties, which can contribute to a feeling of contentment and peace while actually sharpening the senses. Kavalactones produce sedative and muscle relaxant effects. In a randomized, placebo-controlled clinical trial lasting 25 weeks, German researchers found that a standardized kava extract produced anti-anxiety effects in over 100 outpatients with the disorder. They concluded that kava could provide an alternative treatment to tricyclic antidepressants and benzodiazepines. In another recent study, kava consumption was connected with decreased incidence of cancer in a regional population.

Safety: If you are pregnant or nursing, you should avoid using kava. This herb can cause allergic reactions, stomach discomfort, loss of balance, and the inability to focus. Drive with extra caution after having taken kava. Avoid kava if you have a depressive disorder and do not mix it with alcohol, barbiturates or other mood-altering drugs. Be especially careful to avoid taking the tranquilizer Xanax with kava (in one incident, the combination caused a coma). Do not combine kava with valerian root. A hepatitis outbreak has been reported with kava use.

Special Instructions: One study showed that a daily dose of 70 to 210 mg kavalactones produced an anti-anxiety effect. To treat insomnia, a dose of approximately 200 mg of kavalactones taken thirty to sixty minutes prior to retiring has been recommended.

Product Availability: Kava comes in capsules, extracts, dried root and tinctures. Look for products that have a standardized kavalactone content. Kava is often combined with other herbs like hops in formulas designed to treat insomnia or anxiety.

Complementary Agents: hops, chamomile, melatonin

References

Heinze et al. 1994. Pharmacopsychological effects of oxazepam and kava-extract in a visual search paradigm assessed with event-related potentials. *Pharmacopsychiatry* 27(6):224–30.

Kinzler et al. 1991. Effect of a special kava extract in patients with anxiety, tension, and excitation states of non- psychotic genesis. Double blind study with placebos over 4 weeks. *Arzneimittelforschung* 41(6):584–8.

Lindenberg, D. and H. Pitule-Schodel. 1990. D,L-Kavain in comparison with oxazepam in anxiety disorders. A double-blind study of clinical effectiveness. *Forschr Med* 108:49–50,53–54.

Lehmann et al. 1989. The efficacy of Cavain in patients suffering from anxiety. *Pharmacopsychiatry* 22(6):258–62.

Pittler, M. and E. Ernst. 2000. Efficacy of kava extract for treating anxiety: systematic review and meta-analysis. *J Clin Psychopharmacol* 20(1):84–9.

Volz et al. 1997. Kava-kava extract WS 1490 versus placebo in anxiety disorders—a randomized placebo-controlled 25-week outpatient trial. *Pharmacopsychiatry* 30(1):1–5.

Kelp

Overview: Kelp is a broad term that refers to several brown seaweed including over 265 genera and about 2,000 species that grow along the coasts of the Atlantic and Pacific oceans. Kelp is a low-calorie food with a high concentration of minerals. It also boasts a large number of vitamins, amino acids, unsaturated fatty acids, proteins and dietary fiber. It is one of the best natural sources of iodine (also found in iodized salt and some seafood), which is vital for the production of thyroid hormones. An iodine deficiency can lead to an underactive thyroid, which can cause elevated cholesterol, heart problems, obesity and depression. In addition, the fiber content of kelp may have antioxidant, anticoagulant and antitumor properties.

Therapeutic Applications: underactive thyroid, weight loss, hair and nail weakness, circulatory disorders, memory, detoxification, breast cancer, gastric ulcers, liver disorders

Scientific Updates: Kelp may lower blood pressure and cholesterol. It also suppresses the thyroid's ability to absorb radioactive iodine. Kelp also contains mucilage and alginates, which heal mucous membranes. Studies conducted in Japan show a direct correlation between the consumption of algin found in kelp and the prevention of breast cancer. The ability of algin to stimulate the T-cells of the immune system is thought to be responsible for this effect. The micronutrients in kelp also enhance stamina and help to balance hormones. Tests have suggested that it may also have antibiotic properties and may protect the liver from injury. By boosting thyroid function, kelp may increase energy by regulating metabolism and boosting the burning of fat.

Safety: Taking too much kelp for too long can create an overactive thyroid. Daily iodine recommendations are 40 to 50 micrograms for infants, 70 to 120 for children, 150 for adults, 175 for pregnant women and 200 micrograms for lactating women. A fourth teaspoon of iodized salt contains approximately 95 micrograms of iodine. Take all iodine-containing foods into account when deciding kelp intake. Kelp and other seaweed products harvested in industrialized areas can be contaminated with lead, mercury, arsenic and other heavy metals and toxins. Reported side effects include autoimmune thrombocytopenia, dyserythropoiesis and acne-like skin eruptions. Kelp can also be high in sodium and should not be used by anyone following a salt-restricted diet. Do not take kelp if you are pregnant or if suffer from hyperthyroidism. Some doctors also do not recommend consuming kelp when lactating or when suffering from heart problems, but this recommendation is debatable.

Special Instructions: Check labels for iodine content and the place where the kelp was harvested. Various products labeled as kelp aren't always what they seem. Furthermore, the nutrient content of kelp varies between types and numerous other factors (where grown, when picked, etc.).

Product Availability: Kelp can be eaten fresh or dried. It can also be added to soups, stews and salads and is available in tablets, capsules, infusions, teas, powders and liquids.

Complementary Agents: alfalfa, Irish moss, licorice, sarsaparilla, queen of the meadow, vitamin A, vitamin C, bioflavonoids, vitamin E, calcium/magnesium, phosphorus, potassium, zinc, blue-green algae, sea-weed extracts

References

Chiu, K. and A. Fung. 1997. The cardiovascular effects of green beans (Phaseolus aureus), common rue (Ruta graveolens), and kelp (Laminaria japonica) in rats. *Gen Pharmacol* 29(5):859–62.

Funahashi, H. 2000. Breast cancer chemoprevention (tamoxifen, raloxifene, and others). *Nippon Rinsho.* 58 Suppl:587–91.

Maruyama, H., and I. Yamamoto. 1992. Suppression of 125I-uptake in mouse thyroid by seaweed feeding: possible preventative effect of dietary seaweed on internal radiation injury of the thyroid by radioactive iodine. *Kitasato Arch Exp Med* 65(4):209–16.

van Netten et al. 2000. Elemental and radioactive analysis of commercially available sea-weed. *Sci Total Environ* 8:255(1–3):169–75.

Wong et al. 2000. Protective effects of seaweeds against liver injury caused by carbon tetrachloride in rats. *Chemosphere* 41(1–2):173–6.

Kudzu *(Ge-gen)*

Overview: Kudzu is a high-climbing perennial vine. This massive plant has been used for generations by Chinese practitioners for the treatment of fever, diarrhea, headache, neck pain and allergies. Its use for alcohol intoxication has prompted new interest in this herb. It was also recommended for angina. Research suggests that its constituents increase blood flow and oxygenation to heart muscle. It is also a source of phytoestrogens in the form of isoflavones.

Therapeutic Applications: alcohol withdrawal, angina, high blood pressure, fever

Scientific Updates: Chemical compounds found in kudzu root have been linked to improved microcirculation and blood flow. A 1993 study reported that its isoflavones helped to inhibit alcohol cravings and may be of value in treating alcoholism, although a subsequent study disputed this assumption. Kudzu root was also able to absorb heavy metals from water supplies.

Safety: At this writing, there have been no reports of toxicity in humans at recommended dosages. If you are pregnant or are nursing, check with your doctor before using kudzu.

Special Instructions: Chinese practitioners generally suggest taking 9 to

15 grams of kudzu root daily (a large amount). Look for tablets that are standardized. Kudzu tinctures can be used in the amount of 1 to 2 ml taken three times daily.

Product Availability: Kudzu is available in dried root form for tea, capsules and tinctures.

References

Brown et al. 2001. The application of kudzu as a medium for the adsorption of heavy metals from dilute aqueous waste streams. *Bioresour Technol* 78(2):195–201.

Foster, S. 1994. Kudzu root monograph. *Quart Rev Nat Med* Winter:303–8.

Keung, W. and B. Vallee. 1993. Daidzin and daidzein suppress free-choice ethanol intake by Syrian Golden hamsters. *Proc Natl Acad Sci USA* 90:10008–12.

Leung, A. 1996. *Encyclopedia of Common Natural Ingredients Used in Food, Drugs, and Cosmetics, 2nd ed.* New York: John Wiley & Sons. p. 333–6.

Shebek, J. and J. Rindone. 2000. A pilot study exploring the effect of kudzu root on the drinking habits of patients with chronic alcoholism. *J Altern Complement Med* 6(1):45–8.

Lavender *(Lavandula officinalis)*

Overview: Fragrant and lovely, the pale purple lavender flower also contains a variety of medicinal compounds. Lavender grows well in European countries and has been traditionally used for depression, fatigue, headaches and joint diseases. Its popular smell also make it a common addition to soaps and lotions.

Therapeutic Applications: insomnia, anxiety, stress, postpartum perineal support, headaches, perineal healing

Scientific Updates: Essential oil of lavender contains compounds that can tranquilize and promote sleep. One study found that inhaling lavender oil was as effective as some sedatives for sleep. In addition, by prompting faster healing, putting the oil in bath water for perineal pain post childbirth provided more relief than a placebo agent. Lavender can also lower blood pressure in animal studies and it has significant antibacterial and antifungal activity.

Safety: Ingesting the essential oil can cause severe nausea and vomiting. Large doses of lavender can cause drowsiness. External use is considered safe during pregnancy and nursing but the safety of its internal use remains unknown.

Special Instructions: For internal use: Take 1 to 2 ml of tincture twice daily. Make lavender tea by steeping 2 teaspoons of lavender leaves in 1 cup of boiling water for fifteen minutes. Take two to three cups daily. Lavender oil can be added to bathwater or can be used in olive oil as a muscle rub. It can also be placed in an herbal pillow for aromatherapy. Do not use the essential oil internally.

Product Availability: Look for oils that are pure and not made from synthetic lavender. For external applications, lavender comes in oils, creams, lotions etc. For internal applications, it is available as a tea, tincture and capsules.

Complementary Agents: oil of basil, orange peel, passionflower, tea tree oil

References

Buchbauer et al. 1991. Aromatherapy: Evidence for sedative effects of the essential oil of lavender after inhalation. *Z Naturforsch* 46:1067–72.

Dale, A. and S. Cornwell. 1994. The role of lavender oil in relieving perineal discomfort following childbirth: A blind randomized trial. *J Adv Nursing* 19:89–96.

Hardy et al. 1995. Replacement of drug therapy for insomnia by ambient odour. *Lancet* 346:701.

Pattnaik et al. 1997. Antibacterial and antifungal activity of aromatic constituents of essential oils. *Microbios* 89:39–46.

Lemongrass *(Cymbopogon citracus)*

Overview: Chinese medicinal practitioners use lemongrass to treat colds, abdominal distress and headaches. It is also considered a blood cleanser and a good remedy for fevers. Lemongrass helps to expedite the removal of mucus from the body during infections. Today it is commonly used as an essential oil in aromatherapy applications.

Therapeutic Applications: colds, digestive upsets, fever

Scientific Updates: Lemongrass is reputed to reduce mucus discharge in respiratory conditions, due in part to its astringent properties. It has also demonstrated the ability to inhibit the spread of salmonella and has antifungal actions.

Safety: Use in appropriate dosages as directed. Scientists have not established the safety of lemongrass for pregnant or nursing mothers.

Special Instructions: Use only as directed.

Product Availability: Lemongrass is available as an essential oil for aromatherapy applications and also comes as a tea and in capsule form.

Complementary Agents: sage, blessed thistle, marshmallow, mullein, pleurisy root, catnip, chamomile, slippery elm, vitamin C, bioflavonoids, proanthocyanidins, vitamin A

References

Inouye et al. 2000. Inhibitory effect of essential oils on apical growth of Aspergillus fumigatus by vapour contact. *Mycoses* 43(1–2):17–23.

Vinitketkumnuen et al. 1994. Antimutagenicity of lemon grass (Cymbopogon citratus Stapf) to various known mutagens in salmonella mutation assay. *Mutat Res* 341(1):71–5.

Licorice *(Glycyrrhiza glabra, Glycyrrhiza uralensis)*

Overview: Licorice grows in the subtropical climates typical in Greece, Turkey, and Asia Minor. Licorice is an extremely sweet herb that possesses significant antiarthritic and anti-inflammatory properties. These properties are linked to the release of corticosteroid from the adrenal glands. Licorice has been used for adrenal insufficiencies and has recently shown possible treatment benefits for preventing and treating ulcers. It also has demonstrated antiviral and anticancer properties. Perhaps licorice's most popular mainstream use is that of a flavoring in candy, throat lozenges and tobacco.

Therapeutic Applications: arthritis, asthma, bronchitis, canker sores, fibromyalgia, herpes simplex, HIV support, hypoglycemia, indigestion and heartburn, PMS, menopause, peptic ulcer, retinopathy, shingles, coughs

Scientific Updates: Licorice has been the subject of much modern study. Its estrogenic activity has been clearly established. The glycyrrhizin content of licorice stimulates the productions of hormones such as hydrocortisone, which works as efficient anti-inflammatory agents. Glycyrrhizin also stimulates the production of interferon, which boosts immunity. Studies have shown licorice to also possess the ability to counter the effects of two tumor-producing agents. Licorice contains proven anti-inflammatory and anti-allergic properties.

Glycyrrhizin is an anti-inflammatory and inhibits the breakdown of cortisol produced in the adrenal glands. It also has antiviral properties. The flavonoids found in licorice help gastric cells heal and work to protect the liver.

Safety: Licorice supplements that have no glycyrrhizin (DLG) have fewer side effects but are not effective for all applications. Those with glycyrrhizin may increase blood pressure and cause water retention. Long-term intake of licorice at higher than normal dosages can cause these side effects. Prolonged use of glycyrrhizin-containing products should be done with caution and under the supervision of your health care practitioner. Licorice should be avoided if you have high blood pressure, are taking digoxin-based drugs, have liver problems, diabetes, hypokalemia, edema or rapid heartbeat. Taking potassium supplements is recommended while on licorice, but do so only with your doctor's approval. Licorice may lower libido. Some symptoms of toxicity include fatigue, muscle cramping, weakness, edema, headache, impotence, amenorrhea, dark urine and hypertension.

Special Instructions: Look for deglycyrrhizinated licorice (DGL) to use for gastric disorders (especially ulcers). Take one 200 to 300 mg chewable tablet three times daily prior to meals. If you have mouth sores you can mix 200 mg of DGL powder with 1/2 cup of warm water and use it as a gargle. Tinctures of licorice are commonly used in 2 to 5 ml doses three times daily. If you are using licorice for respiratory infections or on the surface of the skin, buy supplements that contain glycyrrhizin. Encapsulated licorice root capsules are commonly used at 4 to 5 grams daily. Licorice teas can be made by boiling 1/2 ounce of root in 1 pint of water for twenty minutes. Two to three cups daily are customary. Apply licorice creams, ointments, or gels directly to herpes sores three to five times daily.

Product Availability: Licorice comes in capsules, chewable tablets, tea, extract, tincture, throat lozenges and syrups, as well as creams and ointments.

Complementary Agents: wild yam, saw palmetto, dong quai, black cohosh, kelp, gotu kola, milk thistle, dandelion, ginger, ginseng, queen of the meadow, sarsaparilla, cramp bark, squaw vine, vitamin E

References

Borrelli, F. and A. Izzo. 2000. The plant kingdom as a source of anti-ulcer remedies. *Phytother Res* 14(8):581–91.

Fujisawa et al. 2000. Glycyrrhizin inhibits the lytic pathway of complement—possible mechanism of its anti-inflammatory effect on liver cells in viral hepatitis. *Microbiol Immunol* 44(9):799–804.

Soma et al. 1994. Effect of glycyrrhizin on cortisol metabolism in humans. *Endocrin Regulations* 28:31–4.

Steinberg et al. 1989. The anticarcinogenic activity of glycyrrhizin: Preliminary clinical trials. *Isr J Dent Sci* 2:153–7.

Tamir et al. 2000. Estrogenic and antiproliferative properties of glabridin from licorice in human breast cancer cells. *Cancer Res* 15:60(20):5704–9.

Tanabe, A. 2000. Steroid hormone- and licorice-induced hypertension. *Nippon Rinsho* 58 Suppl 2:628–32.

Lobelia *(Lobelia inflata)*

Overview: Western herbal practitioners prescribe lobelia for a wide variety of ailments and prize it as a therapeutic herb. Because it has the ability to induce vomiting, it has been the subject of some controversy. Lobelia is an effective and powerful agent for treating bronchitis and asthma because it can dilate the bronchiole tubes. It also acts as a potent relaxant for the central nervous system. It has been associated with tobacco and has been used as a tobacco substitute. It was also recommended to induce sweating and stimulate the expulsion of mucus from the respiratory tract.

Therapeutic Applications: asthma, arthritis, bronchitis, colds, coughs, emphysema, fever, insomnia, lung disease, pleurisy, pneumonia, toothaches, whooping cough, smoking withdrawal

Scientific Updates: In the past, lobelia was approved for use by the FDA as a smoking deterrent in cases of nicotine withdrawal. Lobelia is considered an effective expectorant based on its ability to stimulate the adrenal glands to release corticosteroids, which promote the relaxation of bronchial muscles. Bulgarian scientists recently isolated three new alkaloids from lobelia with significant anti-inflammatory action. Other studies show that lobeline is similar to dextroamphetamine, which may account for lobelia's antidepressant effect. Lobelia is also very rich in chromium.

Safety: Misuse of lobelia can result in vomiting. Lobelia should be taken in exact prescribed dosages. Overdosing can cause serious side effects. Lobelia can cause nausea, diarrhea, headache, dizziness and anxiety. Large doses can cause convulsions or sedation. Lobelia should be avoided by children, and pregnant and nursing women. Lobelia can have a dramatic toxic effect on the nervous system, making it less utilized by herbal practitioners today.

Special Instructions: Use lobelia with caution and only as directed. Do not give it to children unless under the supervision of your health care practitioner. It should not be taken on a daily basis.

Product Availability: Lobelia is available in dried form and in capsules and liquid extracts. Frequently, it is found in combinations containing calamus and mullein designed to break up respiratory congestion.

Complementary Agents: capsicum, garlic, licorice, calamus, skunkweed, comfrey, fenugreek, mullein

References

Philipov et al. 1998. Phytochemical study and antiinflammatory properties of Lobelia lax-iflora L. *Z Naturforsch* 53(5–6):311–7.

Subarnas et al. 1992. An antidepressant principle of Lobelia inflata L. (Campanulaceae). *J Pharm Sci* 81(7):620–21.

Teng et al. 1998. Lobeline displaces [3H]dihydrotetrabenazine binding and releases [3H]dopamine from rat striatal synaptic vesicles: comparison with d-amphetamine. J Neurochem 71(1):258–65.

Lovkova et al. 1996. Medicinal plants—concentrators of chromium. The role of chromium in alkaloid metabolism. *Izv Akad Nauk Ser Biol* (5):552–64.

Lomatium *(Lomatium dissectum)*

Overview: The lomatium plant grows in portions of North America and has been used by Native Americans to treat infections, especially those affecting the respiratory tract. There are over eighty species of this plant with the dissectum being the most therapeutic. Interestingly, lomatium was used to treat the influenza epidemic of 1917, which suggests it has anti-viral properties. It contains tetronic acids and a compound called luteolin, which appears to give it action against invading microorganisms.

Therapeutic Applications: pneumonia, tuberculosis, bronchitis, colds, influenza, sore throats, chest congestion, HIV, viral infections

Scientific Updates: Tetronic acids and a glucoside called luteolin appear to be the main antimicrobial agents found in lomatium root. Lomatium is also terpene rich and is able to stimulate the liquefaction and elimination of mucus from the lungs. Studies also reveal strong antibacterial actions, which interfere with bacterial replication while stimulating immune defenses. It may also have natural blood thinning effects and inhibit the HIV virus.

Special Instructions: Lomatium extracts that have had resins removed are typically used in 1 to 3 ml daily. Tinctures are taken at 1 to 3 ml three times daily. Test a very small amount of tincture first to see if you develop a rash.

Product Availability: Lomatium teas, tinctures and capsules are available. It also comes in topical preparations.

Safety: The resin content of this herb (especially in tincture form) can cause an extensive rash in sensitive individuals. Large doses can also cause nausea and vomiting. Science has not determined the safety of lomatium for pregnant or nursing women. Some members of this genus contain coumarins, which are natural blood thinners. Do not take this herb if you are on any blood thinning drugs.

Complementary Agents: calendula, chamomile, ephedra, eucalyptus, ivy leaf mint oil, thyme

References

Lee et al. 1994. Suksdorfin: an anti-HIV principle from Lomatium suksdorfii, its structure-activity correlation with related coumarins, and synergistic effects with anti-AIDS nucleosides. *Bioorg Med Chem* 2(10):1051–6.

Lee, K. and T. Soine. 1968. Coumarins VII. The coumarins of Lomatium nuttallii. *J Pharm Sci* 57(5):865–8.

McCutcheon et al. 1995. Antiviral screening of British Columbian medicinal plants. *Jour Ethnopharmacol* 1:49(2):101–10.

VanWagenen et al. 1988. Native American food and medicinal plants, Water-soluble constituents of Lomatium dissectum. J Nat Prod. 51(1):136–41.

Marshmallow *(Althaea officinalis)*

Overview: Hippocrates advocated the use of this herb for wound healing. It has the capability of healing inflamed or injured tissue and has demulcent properties, which sooth irritated mucous membranes. The marshmallow grows primarily in marshes, and its roots and leaves are both used for medicinal purposes. It is also calcium-rich and has been used to heal the mucous membranes of the respiratory, gastrointestinal and urinary tracts due to its high mucilage content.

Therapeutic Applications: asthma, colds, coughs, sore throats, Crohn's disease, diarrhea, peptic ulcer, gastrointestinal upset, lung congestion, abrasions, colitis, urinary tract infections

Scientific Updates: Recent laboratory findings disclose that marshmallow contains 286,000 units of vitamin A per pound, which boosts its healing power. The ability of marshmallow to soothe and heal irritated respiratory passages and the intestinal tract is supported by several studies. Marshmallow contains large carbohydrate molecules, which make a slippery substance that can provide a protective covering to irritated mucous membranes. High mucilage herbs have also been associated with positive effects on blood sugar.

Safety: Marshmallow is considered safe and nontoxic; however, look for products from reliable sources to avoid any possibility of contamination.

Special Instructions: You can make marshmallow into a tea by adding its roots and leaves to boiling water and steeping for fifteen minutes. It is also available in extracts and in capsules and tablets. You can take 5 to 6 grams of marshmallow daily. In tincture form 5 to 10 ml used three times daily is recommended. You can also open a capsule and make a slurry by combining the powder with a little water for sore throats and dry coughs.

Product Availability: Marshmallow comes in teas, extracts, tinctures and capsules. It is sometimes added to lozenges to soothe sore throats and inhibit coughs.

Complementary Agents: black cohosh, burdock, slippery elm, mullein, wood betony, chamomile, vitamin E, vitamin A

References

Guevara et al. 1994. The in vitro action of plants on Vibrio cholerae. *Rev Gastroenterol Peru* 14(1):27–31.

Guarnieri et al. 1974. Mucilage of Althaea officinalis. *Farmaco [Prat]* 29(2):83–91.

Nosal'ova et al. 1992. Antitussive action of extracts and polysaccharides of marsh mallow (Althea offcinalis L., var. robusta). *Pharmazie* 47:224–6.

Tomoda et al. 1987. Hypoglycemic activity of twenty plant mucilages and three modified products. *Planta Med* 53:8-12.

Milk Thistle *(Silybum marianum)*

Overview: Milk thistle has a long history of use as an extraordinary liver rejuvenant. Anciently, Dioscorides used it to reverse the poisoning effect of snakebites. Today, European doctors use intravenous applications of milk thistle for mushroom poisoning. The herb has an impressive track record as a liver tonic and protectant. It is the seeds of the milk thistle flower that contain a compound called silymarin. Today people take milk thistle regularly to protect the liver from the effects of heavy metals alcohol, drugs, pesticides and other toxins.

Therapeutic Applications: cirrhosis, hepatitis, diabetes, free radical protection, gallstones, chronic fatigue, jaundice, kidney congestion and disease, liver damage, colitis, poisoning, psoriasis

Scientific Updates: Experiments using silymarin from milk thistle showed that when the herb was given before a deadly mushroom amanita toxin was ingested, it was 100 percent effective in preventing liver toxicity. Studies show that taking milk thistle can result in a pronounced reduction of cholesterol in the bile, which helps to prevent gallbladder disease. Recent studies point to milk thistle as a possible therapy for psoriasis. In addition, the antioxidant activity of a milk thistle seed extract reduced liver damage in test subjects taking potentially harmful psychotic drugs. Other recent studies reveal that silymarin can protect against prostate and skin cancer and better cholesterol profiles.

Safety: Milk thistle is considered safe even for pregnant and nursing women, although no studies have verified this. It may cause a laxative effect in some people although the effect is rare and temporary.

Special Instructions: There is some consensus that taking a reputable standardized milk thistle liquid extract is more effective than capsulized forms of this herb.

Product Availability: Milk thistle is available in tablets, capsules softgels, extracts and tinctures. Teas are not recommended. Look for supplements that are standardized to a 70 to 80 percent silymarin content.

Complementary Agents: dandelion, bioflavonoids, grape seed or pine bark, turmeric, artichoke, schisandra, vitamin E, selenium germanium, marine lipids, essential fatty acids, psyllium

References

Ahmad et al. 1998. Skin cancer chemopreventive effects of a flavonoid antioxidant silymarin are mediated via impairment of receptor tyrosine kinase signaling and perturbation in cell cycle progression. *Biochem Biophys Res Commun* 247(2):294–301.

Cruz et al. 2001. Effects of silymarin on the acute stage of the trinitrobenzenesulphonic acid model of rat colitis. *Planta Med* 67(1):94-6.

Krecman et al. 1998. Silymarin inhibits the development of diet-induced hypercholesterolemia in rats. *Planta Med* 64(2):138–42.

Palasciano Guiseppe et al. 1994. The effect of silymarin on plasma levels of malondialdehyde in patients receiving long-term treatment with psychotropic drugs. *Current Therapeutic Research* 55,5:537–45.

Rastogi et al. 2000. Hepatocurative effect of picroliv and silymarin against aflatoxin B1 induced hepatotoxicity in rats. *Planta Med* 66(8):709–13.

Sharma et al. 2001. Inhibitory effect of silibinin on ligand binding to erbB1 and associated mitogenic signaling, growth, and DNA synthesis in advanced human prostate carcinoma cells. *Mol Carcinog* 30(4):224–36

Mullein *(Verbascum thapsus)*

Overview: It is the leaves and flowers of the mullein plant that are used in medicinal applications. During the Civil War, mullein was used to treat respiratory infections that had irritating dry coughs and chest congestion. Swollen membranes respond to mullein, so it has been used for hay fever. It also has calming properties, so it can be used as a sleep aid. Mullein has reportedly cured warts. It was also recommended for pneumonia and asthma. Like marshmallow, it has a high mucilage content, which was used on the skin to heal burns and rashes.

Therapeutic Applications: common cold, coughs, cramps, ear infections, insomnia, nervousness, upper respiratory problems, sore joints, pain, asthma, bronchitis, chronic obstructive pulmonary disease, sore throat

Scientific Updates: It is thought that the saponins and mucilage contained in mullein enable it to soothe inflammation. In addition, there is some evidence that it may help alleviate pain and promote sleep. Some experts believe that the saponins in mullein are responsible for its expectorant action.

Safety: Mullein is recognized as safe when used as recommended. In certain sensitive people, direct contact with its leaves or flowers can cause dermatitis. There are no known contraindications to its use during pregnancy or nursing.

Special Instructions: Mullein tea can be made by pouring cup of boiling water over 1 to 2 teaspoons of the dried mixture and steeping for fifteen minutes. You can take three to four cups daily. For mullein tincture, take 1 to 4 ml three times daily. For capsulized products, use as directed. Mullein is often used in combinations designed to treat coughs and bronchial congestion. For this reason it may be added to lozenges. You can open a mullein capsule and make a slurry by adding a little water and using it to coat a raw throat.

Product Availability: Mullein comes in lozenges, tinctures, teas, extracts and capsules.

Complementary Agents: horehound, marshmallow, slippery elm, wood betony, lobelia, vitamin E, tea tree oil, aloe vera

References

Grieve, M. A 1971. *Modern Herbal. Vol.* 2. New York: Dover Publications. p. 562–6.

Klimek, B. 1996. 6'-0-apiosyl-verbascoside in the flowers of mullein (Verbascum species). *Acta Pol Pharm* 53(2):137–40.

Romaguera et al. 1985. Occupational dermatitis from Gordolobo (Mullein). *Contact Dermatitis* 12(3):176.

Myrrh Gum *(Commiphora molmol)*

Overview: Myrrh was one of the gifts of the magi as told in the New Testament. It is considered a bitter herb with astringent and antiseptic properties. It has been used to treat mouth disorders and is still prized in certain parts of the world as a precious commodity. The gum resin was also used as a stimulant tonic and is used today as an antiseptic in mouthwashes and dentifrices.

Therapeutic Applications: congestion, indigestion, gas, ulcers, irritable bowel syndrome, ulcerative colitis, high cholesterol, muscle pain, diverticulitis, Crohn's disease, wound healing, sore throats, gingivitis

Scientific Updates: Myrrh apparently works to normalize mucous membrane activity. Because it works this way with the mucous membranes of the stomach lining, it is a valuable digestive aid. Myrrh helps to ensure the proper function of mucous-secreting glands and exerts an antiseptic and antibacterial action at the same time. It has an antiplaque action in the mouth, works as a local anesthetic and also lowers cholesterol levels and blood fats. Some types of myrrh oil can act as muscle relaxants.

Safety: Myrrh has a mild uterine stimulant action and should be avoided in pregnancy. Contact with the oil can cause a rash in sensitive individuals.

Special Instructions: Use the tincture for respiratory infections at a maximum of 5 ml daily diluted in water. Take one 200 mg capsule three times daily. You can make your own gargle by putting 2 ml in one half cup of warm water for sore throats, gum disease and mouth sores. One ml of essential oil in 15 ml of olive oil makes a good chest rub for colds and sore muscles.

Product Availability: Myrrh is available in mouthwashes, capsules, toothpastes, tinctures, essential oil and extracts. You can also buy myrrh resin alone.

Complementary Agents: ginger, fenugreek, catnip, peppermint, fennel, capsicum, acidophilus, saw palmetto, slippery elm digestive enzymes

References

Andersson et al. 1997. Minor components with smooth muscle relaxing properties from scented myrrh (Commiphora guidotti). *Planta Med* 63(3):251–4.

Dolara et al. 1996. Analgesic effects of myrrh. *Nature* 4:379(6560):29.

Dolara et al. 2000. Local anaesthetic, antibacterial and antifungal properties of sesquiterpenes from myrrh. *Planta Med* 66(4):356–8.

Gallo et al. 1999. Allergic contact dermatitis from myrrh. *Contact Dermatitis* 41(4):230–1.

Michie, C. 1991. Frankincense and myrrh as remedies in children. *J R Soc Med* 84(10):602–5.

Noni *(Morinda citrifolia)*

Overview: Virtually every part of this plant has been used for medicinal purposes in the South Pacific for millenia. Noni juice has recently emerged as a valuable therapeutic agent with anti-inflammatory properties, but its leaf and root components are equally beneficial. The noni plant has a wide range of applications due to its adaptogenic properties. Its cancer fighting compounds have recently come to light.

Therapeutic Applications: arthritis, atherosclerosis, bladder infections, boils, bowel disorders, burns, cancer, chronic fatigue syndrome, cold sores, constipation, depression, diabetes, diarrhea, drug addiction, eye inflammations, fever, fractures, gastric ulcers, gingivitis, headaches, hypertension, immune weakness, intestinal parasites, kidney disease, menstrual disorders, pain, respiratory disease, tuberculosis, tumors, wounds

Scientific Updates: Noni contains an impressive array of terpene compounds that have exhibited natural antibiotic activity. The alkaloid content of noni exerts a number of actions, including anti-inflammatory properties. Recent testing has found that certain noni compounds such as damnacanthol have inhibited the growth of precancerous RAS cells. In another study, the ursolic acid found in noni leaves inhibited the growth of a very spreadable form of cancer made up of fibrosarcoma cells. In a 2000 issue of the *International Journal of Oncology*, Korean researchers found that ursolic acid promoted the death of potentially malignant cells. B-sitosterol found in noni juice and leaves can emulsify fats, and in some tests was twenty to thirty times more potent than choline in breaking down cholesterol deposits An article published in a 1999 issue of *Phytotherapy* reported that Noni fruit contains polysaccharides capable of enhancing immune function. The biochemicals found in both noni juice and leaves have also proven themselves to effectively control or kill over six types of infectious bacterial strains including: *E coli*, salmonella, shigella and staphylococcus aureus.

Safety: Extracts of noni are considered safe if used as directed; however, pregnant or nursing women should consult their physician before using any noni derivative. High doses or root extracts may cause constipation. Taking noni supplements with coffee, alcohol or nicotine is not recommended. Noni should be taken on an empty stomach for maximum effectiveness.

Special Instructions: For the leaf, teas have an advantage in that they contain a natural blend of whatever plant or plant parts used. Teas made of leaf or bark constituents need a longer steeping time than regular tea (at least twenty minutes to ensure that the desired plant properties infuse into the water). Water-based sprays can directly target inflamed areas topically or be applied directly to the tongue for absorption. Sprays also have an advantage in that they can be used to make compresses, eye washes, nasal irrigations and gargles. Cold-pressed tablets provide leaf parts in a more convenient form and can be more concentrated, which is ideal when fighting chronic diseases. Taking noni fruit in juice forms provides a complete and natural delivery system to the body with a synergistic and balanced array of enzymes and nutrients in their original form. Freeze-dried fruit juice supplements provide the power of a liquid in the convenience of a capsule, which increases patient compliance, but have to be manufactured and stored properly to ensure potency. Noni juice should be taken on an empty stomach prior to meals in divided doses. Taking one teaspoon before each meal and one teaspoon in the evening is recommended to start. The process of digesting food can interfere with the medicinal value of the alkaloid compounds found in Noni. Because of its strong taste, you may want to dilute it into cranberry or grape juice to make it more palatable.

Product Availability: Noni fruit can be purchased as fruit juice, freeze-dried fruit concentrates, capsulized juice extracts, sprays, soft gels and chewable tablets. Leaf extracts are available in cold-pressed tablets, oils and teas and are sometimes included with other noni plant constituents, which contain a percentage of the fruit, bark, root and seeds for their individual therapeutic properties.

Complementary Agents: cat's claw, *Morinda officinalis*, kava kava, pau d'arco, echinacea, aloe vera, bioflavonoids, selenium, germanium, grape seed extract, proteolytic enzymes, glucosamine, shark cartilage, chondroitin

References

Asuzu et al. 1990. Effects of Morinda lucida leaf extract on Trypanosoma brucei brucei infection in mice. *J Ethnopharmacol* 30(3):307–13.

Choi et al. 2000. Induction of apoptosis by ursolic acid through activation of caspases and down-regulation of c-IAPs in human prostate epithelial cells. *Int J Oncol* 17(3):565–71.

Gupta et al. 1980. Anti-inflammatory and antipyretic activities of B-sitosterol. *Planta Medica* 39:157–163.

Hirazumi A et al 1999. An immunomodulatory polysaccharide-rich substance from the fruit juice of Morinda citrifolia (noni) with antitumour activity. *Phytother Res* 13(5):380–7.

Yoshikawa et al. 1995. Chemical constituents of Chinese natural medicine, morindae radix, the dried roots of morinda officinalis, structures of morindolide and moroffici-naloside. *Chem Pharm Bull* 43(9):1462–5.

Oatstraw *(Avena sativa)*

Overview: Also known as oatgrass, this herb is known for its rich mineral content and its ability to treat osteoporosis, menstrual disorders, urinary tract infections and even hysteria. Tinctures made from oatstraw are used in homeopathic preparations for arthritis, liver ailments and skin disorders. In Europe, oat extracts are used to treat colon disorders and celiac disease. New data suggests that oatstraw has value for celiac disease and is antioxidant rich.

Therapeutic Applications: indigestion, urinary tract infections, osteoporosis, nervous conditions, conditions requiring calcium, celiac disease, menstrual disorders, menopause

Scientific Updates: Oatstraw is an excellent natural source of calcium and magnesium. It is considered a superior plant source of magnesium. New studies point to the glutathione content of its seeds; glutathione actually increases the effect and longevity of some antioxidants in the body. The discovery of phytosterols in oatstraw confirm its traditional use for menstrual disorders and menopause.

Safety: Oatstraw has no known toxicity; however, allergic reactions can occur with extract products in some sensitive individuals. Pregnant or nursing women should consult a physician before use.

Special Instructions: To be considered of good quality, oatstraw should be a rich, green color and have a characteristic odor. Oatstraw tea is considered superior to capsulized supplements because of its rapid assimilation.

Product Availability: Oatstraw comes in teas, extracts, capsules, powders and tinctures. It is sometimes added to green drink formulas for detoxification.

Complementary Agents: plantain, marshmallow, alfalfa, barley grass, red clover, calcium/magnesium

References

Emmons et al. 1999. Antioxidant capacity of oat (Avena sativa L.) extracts. In vitro antioxidant activity and contents of phenolic and tocol antioxidants. *J Agric Food Chem* 47(12):4894–8.

Hoffenberg et al. 2000. A trial of oats in children with newly diagnosed celiac disease. *J Pediatr* 137(3):361–6.

Pazzaglia et al. 2000. Allergic contact dermatitis due to avena extract. *Contact Dermatitis* 42(6):364.

Trojanowska et al. 2000. Biosynthesis of avenacins and phytosterols in roots of Avena sativa cv. Image. *Phytochemistry* 54(2):153–64.

Zachariah et al. 2000. Isolation, purification, and characterization of glutathione S-transferase from oat (Avena sativa) seedlings. *J Protein Chem* 19(6):425–30.

Oregon Grape *(Berberis aquifolium)*

Overview: Oregon grape is another berberine-containing herb used to treat infection. Its ability to contribute to blood cleansing makes it a favorite choice for the treatment of skin disorders. It is also considered a glandular tonic and was traditionally used by Native Americans to treat jaundice, diarrhea, fever and infections of all kinds.

Therapeutic Applications: acne, anemia, blood purification, fever, indigestion, immune system, infections, eczema, jaundice, liver disorders, psoriasis, skin ailments, staph infections, vaginal yeast infections, conjunctivitis/blepharitis, parasites, poor digestion, urinary tract infections

Scientific Updates: Laboratory studies have confirmed that Oregon grape has a bacteriocidal effect against strep infections similar to that of goldenseal. Studies show that an ointment of Oregon grape can effectively treat skin infections. In other scientific studies, whole Oregon grape extracts reduced inflammation and stimulated the activity of white blood cells. The berberine contained in this herb has also been shown to effectively treat diarrhea in people infected with *E. coli*. Berberine also prevents bacteria from attaching to human cells, which may explain why it is so helpful with urinary tract infections.

Safety: Berberine-containing herbs should not be used for long periods of time or in large dosages. They are not recommended for pregnant or nursing women. Berberine alone has been reported to interfere with normal bilirubin metabolism in infants; therefore, it should not be used by nursing women.

Special Instructions: Oregon grape tea can be made by boiling 1 to 3 teaspoons of the root in 2 cups of water for twenty minutes. Strain and cool the mixture and up to 3 cups daily can be taken. You can also take 3 ml of tincture three times daily.

Product Availability: Look for standardized extracts containing 5 to 10 percent alkaloids, which can provide 500 mg of berberine daily. For topical applications, look for a 10 percent extract ointment and apply three or more times daily for inflammatory skin diseases like psoriasis.

Complementary Agents: goldenseal, barberry, garlic, echinacea, myrrh, dandelion, burdock, capsicum, vitamin A, vitamin C, bioflavonoids, acidophilus, blue-green algae

References

Berberine. 2000. *Altern Med Rev* 5(2):175–7.

Kumazawa et al. 1984. Activation of peritoneal macrophages by berberine-type alkaloids in terms of induction of cytostatic activity. *Int J Immunopharmacol* 6:587–92.

Rabbani et al. 1987. Randomized controlled trial of berberine sulfate therapy for diarrhea due to enterotoxigenic Escherichia coli and Vibrio cholerae. *J Infect Dis* 155(5):979–84.

Sun et al. 1988. Berberine sulfate blocks adherence of Streptococcus pyogenes to epithelial cells, fibronectin, and hexadecane. *Antimicrob Agents Chemother* 32(9):1370–74.

Wiesenauer, M. and R. Lüdtke. 1996. Mahonia aquifolium in patients with psoriasis vulgaris—an intraindividual study. *Phytomed* 3:231–35.

Papaya *(Papaya Puama)*

Overview: Papayas are small fruits that grow in tropical climates. A compound called papain comes from green papayas and provides a combination of valuable enzymes that are actually used in meat tenderizers due to their ability to break down protein. When taken as a medicine, papain boosts the digestion of protein in the stomach. Used on the skin, it can promote tissue healing and help to remove dead skin. Traditional applications of papaya include: gastrointestinal problems, psoriasis and wound healing.

Therapeutic Applications: indigestion, ulcers, cancer, constipation, pancreatic insufficiency, skin problems, poisonous bites, yeast infections, diabetes, Alzheimer's disease

Scientific Updates: Studies have found papain to be valuable for foot ulcers and for treating yeast infections, especially when combined with standard antifungal drugs. Asian researchers confirmed the high antioxidant action of fermented papaya. Other studies suggest that papaya may help to prevent cancer by programming malignant cells to die. It may also benefit Alzheimer's, diabetes and other degenerative diseases associated with free radical damage. Some studies suggest its use for colon cancer. Papaya is rich in vitamin C, fiber, folic acid, and beta-carotene.

Safety: Papaya fruit is considered safe. Isolated papain supplements should not be taken by pregnant women or people on blood thinning drugs. Papain may also cause allergic reactions in sensitive individuals.

Special Instructions: For indigestion use chewable papaya tablets fifteen minutes prior to eating.

Product Availability: Papaya is sold in capsules, teas and chewable tablets. It is commonly added to digestive enzyme formulas.

References

Beers, E.P. and B.J. Woffenden. 2000. Plant proteolytic enzymes: possible roles during programmed cell death. *Plant Mol Biol* 44(3):399–415.

Giordani et al. 1997. A synergistic effect of Carica papaya latex sap and fluconazole on Candida albicans growth. *Mycoses* 40(11-12):429–37.

Imao et al. 1998. Free radical scavenging activity of fermented papaya preparation and its effect on lipid peroxide level and superoxide dismutase activity in iron-induced epileptic foci of rats. *Biochem Mol Biol Int* 45(1):11–23.

Otuka et al. 1996. The use of papain in plantar ulcers. *Rev Bras Enferm* 49(2):207–14.

Popiela et al. 2000. Enzyme therapy in patients with advanced colorectal cancer. *Przegl Lek* 57 Suppl 5:138–9.

Parsley *(Petroselinum sativum)*

Overview: Much more than just a garnish, parsley supplies chlorophyll, restores the urinary tract, and increases lactation. It can also alleviate the bad breath caused by eating garlic. It was traditionally used to decrease water retention, and reduce high blood pressure. Parsley seeds were also used to stimulate uterine contractions, and the leaf was applied to gastrointestinal disorders, flatulence, urinary tract infections and jaundice. Topical forms of parsley were used to ease muscle pain and heal wounds.

Therapeutic Applications: bedwetting, bladder infections, blood disorders, diabetes, edema, gallstones, halitosis, jaundice, kidney disease, kidney stones, prostate disorders, water retention, indigestion, heartburn, menstrual ailments

Scientific Updates: Studies have shown that in comparison to citrus juices, parsley contains three times more vitamin C gram per gram. Parsley's high chlorophyll content can freshen breath even after eating garlic and onions. Recent studies have found parsley to be beneficial for high blood pressure, and Hungarian scientists have confirmed its high antioxidant action due to its rich content of flavonoids. Constituents of the essential oil are known to stimulate the uterus, increase urination, reduce inflammation of the urinary tract and to kill microbes. It is also thought that parsley can kill microorganisms and tone the uterus while acting as a liver tonic and stimulating urination. A new study suggests that parsley leaf oil may inhibit the growth of tumors.

Safety: Parsley leaves and roots are considered safe, however the seeds or essential oil of the seeds are potentially toxic. Parsley seed oil should not be used medicinally, and even the leaves and roots should not be taken by pregnant or nursing women, people with kidney disease or those with very fair skin. Large doses of the seeds or its essential oil can cause nausea, headache, light sensitivity and long-term damage to the kidney and the liver.

Special Instructions: Eating fresh parsley leaves after a spicy meal can help to prevent halitosis. Parsley leaf tea is also recommended when treating urinary tract infections.

Product Availability: Parsley supplements are available in the fresh leaf, capsules, liquid extracts, essential oils and teas. It is often added to formulas containing garlic or ones designed to treat the urinary tract and for detoxification and indigestion.

Complementary Agents: buchu, cornsilk, alfalfa, uva ursi, juniper berry, cranberry, marshmallow, kelp, saw palmetto, garlic, vitamin C, bioflavonoids, vitamin A, vitamin E, zinc, proanthocyanidins, bee pollen

References

Ali-Shtayeh et al. 2000. Ethnobotanical survey in the Palestinian area: a classification of the healing potential of medicinal plants. *J Ethnopharmacol* 73(1–2):221–32.

Fejes S et al. 1998. Investigation of the in vitro antioxidant effect of Petroselinum crispum (Mill.) Nym. ex A. W. Hill*Acta Pharm Hung* 68(3):150–6.

Zheng et al. 1992. Inhibition of benzo[a]pyrene-induced tumorigenesis by myristicin, a volatile aroma constituent of parsley leaf oil. *Carcinogenesis* 13(10):1921–3.

Ziyyat A et al. 1997. Phytotherapy of hypertension and diabetes in oriental. *Morocco J Ethnopharmacol* 58(1):45–54.

Passionflower *(Passiflora incarnata)*

Overview: Used as an effective nervous-system calmant in Europe, passionflower is recommended for anyone trying to get off pharmaceutical sleeping pills. It is also suggested for eye inflammations and hyperactivity. Interestingly, passionflower seeds have been identified with very ancient cultures and have a long history of use as a botanical hypnotic. In topical form, passionflower was used to heal cuts and burns. European practitioners consider passionflower and valerian root to be the two most effective herbal relaxants and sedatives.

Therapeutic Applications: alcoholism, anxiety, eye inflammations, insomnia, nervousness, headaches, ADHD, hypertension, cardiovascular disease, asthma, hormonal imbalances, stress, nervous indigestion, hemorrhoids (topically)

Scientific Updates: Recent studies confirm the presence of a compound called chrysin in passionflower that works as an anticonvulsant and muscle relaxant compared to Valium for its efficacy. Other studies have found that extracts of passionflower can treat anxiety disorders and can promote longer periods of sleep. Its rich alkaloid content is thought to be responsible for these effects. It is also possible that passionflower contains low levels of serotonin, a neurotransmitter that naturally calms the brain, thus achieving relaxation. It has also shown the ability to expand the coronary arteries of the heart, thereby decreasing blood pressure. Passionflower has also been recommended for ADHD due to its calming effect.

Product Availability: You can purchase passionflower as a liquid extract, capsules, teas and tinctures. You will often see it combined with other nervine herbs like valerian or with melatonin for insomnia. It is also added to combinations designed to treat stress, depression or anxiety disorders.

Safety: If taken as directed, passionflower is considered relatively safe and nonhabit forming. Some reports of upset stomach have been cited. It should not be used by pregnant or nursing women. Large doses of passionflower can cause toxicity.

Complementary Agents: valerian root, hops, capsicum, peppermint, chamomile, melatonin, GABA, calcium/ magnesium

References

Berdonces, J.L. 2001. Attention deficit and infantile hyperactivity. *Rev Enferm* 24(1):11–4.

Bourin et al. 1997. A combination of plant extracts in the treatment of outpatients with adjustment disorder with anxious mood: controlled study versus placebo. *Fundam Clin Pharmacol* 11(2):127–32

Gerhard et al. 1991. Acute sedative effect of a herbal relaxation tablet as compared to that of bromazepam. *Schweiz Rundsch Med Prax* 27:80(52):1481–6.

Medina et al. 1990. Chrysin (5,7-di-OH-flavone), a naturally-occurring ligand for benzodiazepine receptors, with anticonvulsant properties. *Biochem Pharmacol* 40(10):2227–31.

Soulimani et al. 1997. Behavioural effects of Passiflora incarnata L. and its indole alkaloid and flavonoid derivatives and maltol in the mouse. *J Ethnopharmacol* 57(1):11–20.

Pleurisy Root *(Asclepias tuberosa)*

Overview: Traditionally used to treat any respiratory disorder, pleurisy root has the ability to expedite the removal of lung mucus. It is one of nature's best expectorants and has a long history of use to liquify mucus and expel it from the body. Used in folk medicine as a decoction, it was administered for lung congestion typically seen in diseases like bronchitis.

Therapeutic Applications: allergies, asthma, bronchitis, emphysema, pneumonia, tuberculosis, cough, sore throat, colds, tuberculosis

Scientific Updates: Pleurisy root specifically targets the lungs and stimulates the removal of thick mucus. It helps to mitigate pain and inflammation typical of lung infections. The reputation of pleurisy root as an excellent therapeutic for lung ailments extends back for several centuries. Earlier in the century, it was considered a primary expectorant. The glycosides in this herb are thought to thin mucus for easier expulsion. Recently, several new glycoside compounds have been discovered in pleurisy root.

Safety: The safety of pleurisy root in pregnant or nursing women has not been established. Check with your doctor before combining it with any over-the-counter or prescription drug. Use dosages only as directed.

Special Instructions: Combining the use of pleurisy root with mullein may make for a more powerful lung decongestant.

Product Availability: Pleurisy root is available in capsules, extracts, tinctures and teas.

Complementary Agents: slippery elm, wild cherry bark, sage, thyme, mullein, fenugreek, capsicum, marshmallow, vitamin C, bioflavonoids, vitamin A, calcium/magnesium, bee pollen, acidophilus

References

Abe, F. and T. Yamauchi. 2000. Pregnane glycosides from the roots of Asclepias tuberosa. *Chem Pharm Bull (Tokyo)* 48(7):1017–22.

Pagani, F. 1975. Phyto-constituents of Asclepias tuberosa L. (Asclepiadaceae). *Boll Chim Farm* 114(8):450–6.

Pau d'Arco/Taheebo (Tabebuia avellandedae)

Overview: Pau d'arco (also known as taheebo) is relatively new to Western herbalists. It is harvested from the very hard bark of the lapacho tree in South America. Pau d'arco has been linked to cancer cures and at one time was investigated by the National Cancer Institute for its anticancer properties. Today it continues to be used for malignancies, especially leukemia, and is also prescribed for herpes, diabetes, arthritis and hypoglycemia. It is under current study for its possible value in treating AIDS.

Therapeutic Applications: AIDS, blood disorders, candida, infections, liver disease, pain (arthritis), prostate disorders, psoriasis, ringworm, ulcers, anemia, cancer (especially leukemia), diabetes, herpes, hypoglycemia, lupus, parasites, skin diseases (including cancer), tumors, sexually transmitted diseases (STDs) and yeast infections

Scientific Updates: Some of the chemical constituents of pau d'arco have shown the ability to suppress tumor formation. Some researchers believe that the lapacho content of pau d'arco is one of the most important antitumor agents in the world. Pau d'arco has also proven its antibacterial and antiviral properties and may help to treat psoriasis.

Safety: In unusual cases, mild nausea or a laxative effect has occurred. Rotating pau d'arco therapy with mataike tea is sometimes advised. Do not take lapacho compounds isolated from pau d'arco; instead use the whole herb. Some animal studies of long-term, high-dose consumption of lapachol have shown that it may reduction of red blood cells.

Special Instructions: Taking this herb in tea form is recommended, especially for recurring yeast infections.

Product Availability: Pau d'arco is available as a tincture, in capsules and as dried bark. Look for products with standardized lapachal content that use the whole root.

Complementary Agents: licorice, garlic, echinacea, goldenseal, black walnut, cat's claw, alfalfa, burdock, kelp, milk thistle, dandelion, maitake, Oregon grape, yellow dock, yerba maté

References
de Santana et al. 1968. Antitumoral and toxicological properties of extracts of bark and

various wood components of Pau d'arco (Tabebuia avellanedae). *Rev Inst Antibiot (Recife)* 8(1):89–94.

Dinnen, R. and K. Ebisuzaki. 1997. The search for novel anticancer agents: a differentiation-based assay and analysis of a folklore product. *Anticancer Res* 17(2A):1027–33.

Muller et al. 1999. Potential antipsoriatic agents: lapacho compounds as potent inhibitors of HaCaT cell growth. *J Nat Prod* 62(8):1134–6.

Pinto et al. 2000. Chemical reactivity studies with naphthoquinones from Tabebuia with anti-trypanosomal efficacy. *Arzneimittelforschung* 50(12):1120–8.

Ueda et al. 1994. Production of anti-tumour-promoting furanonaphthoquinones in Tabebuia avellanedae cell cultures. *Phytochemistry* 36(2):323–5.

Peppermint *(Mentha piperita)*

Overview: Peppermint is one the most popular herbal teas in America and has a wide array of pleasant and therapeutic properties. Used for flavoring and for its menthol content, it has both stimulant and antispasmodic actions. Traditionally, it was used for indigestion, gas, heartburn, diarrhea, respiratory and gallbladder disease, and intestinal cramping. Peppermint tea is also considered a popular remedy for morning sickness.

Therapeutic Applications: colds, sinusitis, bronchitis, diarrhea, gastritis, enteritis, indigestion, nausea, intestinal gas, bloating, gripping, colitis, heartburn, irritable bowel syndrome, gallstones, stomach spasms, ulcers, vomiting, loss of appetite, gum disease, tension headache

Scientific Updates: Today peppermint is recognized for its soothing action on the stomach and intestines. It works as an antispasmodic, which relieves nausea and other stomach maladies. Peppermint relaxes the muscles of the digestive tract and stimulates bile flow, which facilitates more efficient digestion. A 1995 double-blind, placebo-controlled study found that essential oil of peppermint rubbed into the forehead may relieve tension headaches. Other data suggest that enteric-coated peppermint oil formulations can reduce the symptoms of irritable bowel syndrome. In another study, scientists reported that peppermint oil may help to prevent post-surgical nausea. Applied to the skin, the menthol contained in peppermint oil dilates blood vessels and relaxes muscles. Peppermint also has antimicrobial and anti-inflammatory actions.

Safety: Oil of peppermint can be irritating to mucous membranes if used excessively. Use with caution if pregnant or breast feeding. Do not give peppermint preparations in large doses to infants for colic or young children. The volatile oils contained in peppermint can cause liver damage. If you have gallstones, you may experience some intestinal discomfort. When used on the skin, the oil may cause irritation. Peppermint oil may also cause an asthma-like attack if applied directly around the nose of an infant or small child. Taking peppermint in capsule form that has not be coated enterically may cause a burning sensation in the stomach may occur.

Special Instructions: If using peppermint for irritable bowel syndrome, make sure to purchase enteric coated capsules, so the oil will be released in the lower bowel.

Product Availability: Peppermint is available as a tea, in dried leaf form, enteric capsules, as an essential oil and as an herbal oil. You can also purchase it in liquid extracts and softgels. It is often combined with ginger and digestive enzymes in gastrointestinal formulas.

Complementary Agents: catnip, fennel, ginger, myrrh, capsicum, saw palmetto, calcium carbonate, digestive enzymes

References

Göbel et al. 1995. Essential plant oils and headache mechanisms. *Phytomedicine* 2(2):93–102.

Kline et al. 2001. Enteric-coated, pH-dependent peppermint oil capsules for the treatment of irritable bowel syndrome in children. *J Pediatr* 138(1):125–8.

Liu J et al. 1997. Enteric-coated peppermint-oil capsules in the treatment of irritable bowel syndrome: a prospective, randomized trial. *J Gastroenterol* 32(6):765–68.

Pittler, M. and E. Ernst. 1998. Peppermint oil for irritable bowel syndrome: a critical review and metaanalysis. *Am J Gastroenterol* 93(7):1131–35.

Tate, S. 1997. Peppermint oil: a treatment for postoperative nausea. *J Adv Nurs* 26(3):543–49.

Pumpkin Seed *(Cucurbita pepo)*

Overview: The pumpkin has long been a symbol of health in China. In modern times its seeds have been found to have significant antiparasitic properties and are routinely used to rejuvenate the prostate gland. As a rich source of zinc, pumpkin seed is highly recommended for the male reproductive system. Pumpkin seed is highly nutritional.

Therapeutic Applications: prostate disorders, intestinal parasites, worms, male infertility

Scientific Updates: Some scientific studies have found that oil constituents of pumpkin seed combined with saw palmetto can effectively treated an enlarged prostate gland. Pumpkin seed contains plant sterols, which help to balance hormones. Pumpkin seed is also thought to be a natural diuretic. The seed contains a rare amino acid called myosin, which is the primary protein constituent of muscles and is rich in fatty acids.

Safety: Take only as directed. Do not take pumpkin seed if pregnant or nursing unless advised by your doctor.

Special Instructions: Taking pumpkin seed for prostate disorders works more effectively when combined with saw palmetto, pygeum and soy isoflavones.

Product Availability: While this herb is available as a single supplement, it works best when combined with other antiparasitic herbs or in formulas designed to treat the prostate. Eating roasted pumpkin seeds is also recommended.

Complementary Agents: saw palmetto, pygeum, kelp, garlic, black walnut, red clover, cascara sagrada, quassia, buckthorn, acidophilus, bee pollen, bee propolis, soy isoflavones, B-complex, vitamin E, bioflavonoids, zinc

References

Carbin et al. 1990. Treatment of benign prostatic hyperplasia with phytosterols. *Br J Urol* 66(6):639–41.

Murkovic et al. 1996. Variability of fatty acid content in pumpkin seeds (Cucurbita pepo L.). *Z Lebensm Unters Forsch* 203(3):216–9.

Reindl et al. 2000. Allergy caused by ingestion of zucchini (Cucurbita pepo): characterization of allergens and cross-reactivity to pollen and other foods. *J Allergy Clin Immunol* 106(2):379–85.

Pygeum *(Pygeum africanum)*

Overview: Pygeum is an evergreen tree that grows in the mountainous regions of central and southern Africa. The bark was used to treat urinary disorders. Subsequent modern investigation has found that components in Pygeum bark do indeed benefit BPH (benign prostate hyperplasia) and other diseases of the prostate. Like pumpkin seed, pygeum contains phytosterols including one called beta-sitosterol that has significant anti-inflammatory action.

Therapeutic Applications: prostatitis, BPH, prostate cancer, male urinary disorders, incontinence

Scientific Updates: The phytosterols in pygeum work to inhibit the production of inflammatory prostaglandins that can settle in prostate tissue causing (BPH). In addition, the terpenes found in this herb block swelling. Other constituents balance hormones and inhibit the accumulation of toxins and cholesterol in the prostate gland. By so doing, the negative effects of testosterone and its related hormones are decreased in the prostate. It also appears to positively effect bladder muscle, which could benefit some types of incontinence.

Safety: Side effects are rare. There are reports of mild gastrointestinal upset. Because the primary application of this herb is for prostate disorders, pregnant or nursing women should not take pygeum.

Special Instructions: Look for products with a lipophilic content standardized to 13 percent total sterols. The typical dose is between 50 to 100 mg two times daily. Pygeum needs to be taken for at least three to six months to be effective. If you have BPH, stay in close contact with your doctor, and inform him or her of your pygeum treatments.

Product Availability: Pygeum is available as a single supplement in capsules and liquid extracts. It is, however, most often included in prostate supportive formulas that contain saw palmetto and pumpkin seed.

Complementary Agents: saw palmetto, pumpkin seed, zinc, bee pollen, soy isoflavones

References
Chen et al. 1999. Effects of Unilateral Ischemia on the Contractile Response of the Bladder: Protective Effect of Tadenan (Pygeum africanum Extract). *Mol Urol* 3(1):5–10.

McQueen, C. and P. Bryant. 2001. Pygeum. *Am J Health Syst Pharm* 15:58(2):120–3.

Szolnoki et al. 2001. The effect of Pygeum africanum on fibroblast growth factor (FGF) and transforming growth factor beta (TGF beta 1/LAP) expression in animal model. *Acta Microbiol Immunol Hung* 48(1):1–9.

Wilt et al. 2000. Phytotherapy for benign prostatic hyperplasia. *Public Health Nutr* 3(4A):459–72.

Red Clover *(Trifolium pratense)*

Overview: Red clover, a sweet herb and relative of white clover, is an excellent blood purifier and antibiotic. Its isoflavone content makes it particularly valuable for women's disorders. Traditionally, it was used for skin eruptions and gained notoriety in the early 20th century when it became part of the famous Hoxsey formula of special herbs selected for their ability to fight cancer. The fact that red clover has been successfully used in Australia (Promensel™) for a number of gynecological problems has sparked new interest in the plant for women's ailments.

Therapeutic Applications: menstrual disorders, menopause, endometriosis, fibrocystic disease, acne, bladder infections, boils, bronchitis, infertility, cancer, leukemia, liver disorders, nervous conditions, psoriasis, skin ailments (eczema), tumors

Scientific Updates: Clinical studies have found that red clover contains antibiotic properties against several bacteria, including those that cause tuberculosis. Scientists have also discovered that red clover contains molybdenum, a trace element that is now recognized as essential in clearing the body of nitrogenous waste material. Ounce for ounce red clover has more isoflavones than soy, making it a valuable phytoestrogen for female conditions caused by hormonal imbalance. One isoflavone called genistein may help prevent cancer.

Safety: Nonfermented red clover is considered generally safe. The fermented versions, however, should be avoided. Allergic reactions can occur in sensitive individuals who come in contact with dried red clover flowers. Red clover should not be taken by anyone on anticoagulant drugs such as Coumadin (warfarin). Pregnant or nursing women should not use red clover, neither should children under 10 years of age. No interactions have been reported from combining standard HRT (hormonal replacement therapy) or oral contraceptives with red clover, but check with your health care provider anyway. If you have had breast cancer or are undergoing treatment, check with your doctor before taking any supplement.

Special Instructions: Red clover tea can be made by placing 1 cup of boiling water over 3 teaspoons of dried red clover flowers and steeping for fifteen minutes. Taking three cups daily is customary. Red clover is also available in capsule or tablet form, and the daily dosage can vary from 1,000 to 3,000 mg daily. Tinctures are usually taken in 2 to 4 ml doses three times daily. Dried red clover can be added to salads or other foods. You may not see any noticeable difference until you've been on the supplement for 3 to 6 weeks; and if you stop, benefits will cease.

Product Availability: Red clover comes in teas, capsules, extracts and tinctures and is often added to women's formulas that contain soy isoflavones or other phytoestrogenic herbs.

Complementary Agents: soy isoflavones, natural progesterone, black cohosh, licorice, parsley sarsaparilla, alfalfa

References

A dietary supplement derived from red clover, called P-081, significantly increased HDL (good) cholesterol levels in postmenopausal women, according to results of a study. 1998. New York: *Reuters Health*

Chiechi, L.M. 1999. Dietary phytoestrogens in the prevention of long-term postmenopausal diseases. Department of Obstetrics and Gynaecology III, University of Bari, Italy. *International Journal of Gynaecology and Obstetrics* 67(1):39–40.

Nestel et al. 1999. Isoflavones from red clover improve systemic arterial compliance but not plasma lipids in menopausal women. *Journal of Clinical Endocrinology Metabolism* 84(3):895–8.

Red Raspberry *(Rubus idaeus)*

Overview: Known for its delicious berries, the red raspberry bush can also help to ease female discomforts while strengthening uterine muscle. It can also promote tissue healing and healthy skin, bones and teeth. Traditionally, red raspberry was looked to for excessive menstrual flow (menorrhagia) and to prepare the uterus for delivery during pregnancy.

Therapeutic Applications: after-birth pains, bowel disorders, childbirth, diarrhea, digestive problems, female complaints, fever, flu, heart disease, lactation, menstrual irregularities, miscarriage, morning sickness, mouth sores, nausea, common cold/sore throat, postpartum support

Scientific Updates: Research has found that red raspberry leaf is rich in antioxidants, and that it may act to tone uterine muscles. It is also thought that red raspberry may build the tissue of the cervix to prevent tearing during delivery, although these constituents have not been identified. Raspberry leaves are rich in tannins, which may explain its use for acute diarrhea.

Safety: While mild doses are recommended during pregnancy, excessive amounts should be avoided. Raspberry may cause loose stools and mild nausea.

Special Instructions: Raspberry leaf tea can be made by placing 1 cup of boiling water over 2 teaspoons of the dried herb and steeping for ten to fifteen minutes. Two to three cups daily is customary. Tinctures are typically used in 4 to 8 ml doses taken three times daily.

Product Availability: Taking red raspberry in tea form is a favorite. It is also available in tinctures, extracts and capsules.

Complementary Agents: licorice, dong quai, saw palmetto, licorice, cramp bark, damiana, queen of the meadow, squaw vine, sarsaparilla, black cohosh, B-complex, folic acid, vitamin E, calcium/magnesium, primrose oil

References

Aoussat, A. and A. Latrasse. 2000. Antimicrobial effects of Finnish plant extracts containing flavonoids and other phenolic compounds. *Int J Food Microbiol* 25:56(1):3–12.

McFarlin et al. 1999. A national survey of herbal preparation use by nurse-midwives for labor stimulation. Review of the literature and recommendations for practice. *J Nurse Midwifery* 44(3):205–16.

Wang, S. and H. Lin. 2000. Antioxidant activity in fruits and leaves of blackberry, raspberry, and strawberry varies with cultivar and developmental stage. *J Agric Food Chem* 48(2):140–6.

Red Sage (Salvia officinalis)

Overview: Red sage has been associated with wisdom and longevity for millennia. It has traditionally been used for menstrual disorders, to reduce night sweats and as a natural mouth deodorizer. The volatile oils in red sage have antiseptic and astringent properties and are also used to help dry up milk supplies when a woman wishes to stop breastfeeding.

Therapeutic Applications: coughs, depression, fever, diabetes, digestive disorders, liver aliments, lactation inhibitor, menstrual pain, mouth sores, nausea, nervous conditions, night sweats, sores, sore throat, worms, (failing) memory

Scientific Updates: The volatile oils and tannins in red sage are responsible for its ability to stop excessive perspiration. The oils also have an antiseptic and astringent property, which makes them useful in the healing of sores and irritations. A recent study confirmed the anti-inflammatory action of red sage in topical preparations. The ursolic content of this herb has also shown antitumor properties. Red sage also acts as a powerful antioxidant and boosts circulation. Its estrogenic properties may explain its believed ability to dry up breast milk.

Safety: Avoid red sage during pregnancy while nursing and in cases of epilepsy. Red sage contains a compound called thujone, which can trigger seizures in epileptics.

Special Instructions: For a compress, soak a cotton cloth in red sage tea and apply to specific area. Teas can also be used as a gargle for sore throats, mouth sores and gum disease. Tinctures are recommended for menstrual problems.

Product Availability: Red sage comes in tea form, tinctures, essential oil, capsules and can be included in creams and ointments.

Complementary Agents: capsicum, dandelion, garlic, yellow dock, quassia, milk thistle, cascara sagrada, black walnut, acidophilus, noni, blue-green algae, proanthocyanidins, vitamin C, vitamin A, B-complex, calcium/magnesium

References

Baricevic et al. 2001. Topical anti-inflammatory activity of Salvia officinalis L. leaves: the relevance of ursolic acid. *J Ethnopharmacol* 75(2–3):125–132.

Hromadkova et al. 1999. Comparison of classical and ultrasound-assisted extraction of polysaccharides from Salvia officinalis L. *Ultrason Sonochem* 5(4):163–8.

Lu, Y. and L. Foo. 2000. Flavonoid and phenolic glycosides from Salvia officinalis. *Phytochemistry* 55(3):263–7.

Salisova et al. 1997. Comparison of conventional and ultrasonically assisted extractions of pharmaceutically active compounds from Salvia officinalis. *Ultrason Sonochem* 4(2):131–4.

Rose Hips *(Rosa species)*

Overview: A rose hip, the fleshy fruit of a rose blossom, is an unusually rich source of vitamin C. Rose hips were used in England during World War II to offset the shortage of citrus fruits and prevent scurvy. Rose hips contain sixty times more vitamin C than lemons.

Therapeutic Applications: arteriosclerosis, bladder infections, blood purifier, cancer, circulatory insufficiencies, colds, contagious diseases, fever, flu, infections, PMS, sore throat, stress, (any inflammatory condition)

Scientific Updates: Linus Pauling's research on vitamin C literally put rose hips on the map as a therapeutic agent. His research points to daily doses to prevent all kinds of illness and to promote longevity. Rose hips provide a superior, natural source of vitamin C, which has been linked to the prevention and cure of certain cancers. Its ability to lower blood serum cholesterol and to shorten the duration of a cold is well supported by scientific data. New studies point to its ability to fight wrinkles and protect skin tissue when applied topically even when exposed to ultraviolet light.

Safety: Vitamin C can be taken in high doses, although stomach upset and diarrhea may occur in some cases. People who have trouble with kidney stones should consult their physicians before taking supplemental doses of vitamin C. Taking calcium/magnesium with vitamin C increases its assimilation. Very large doses have recently been linked to the possible development of malignant cells.

Special Instructions: You can add rose hip oil to creams and use for skin inflammations or for cosmetic purposes. Combining it with vitamin E enhances its action.

Product Availability: You can purchase rose hips as dried leaves, essential oil, syrups, powders, capsules, in fruit drinks and as teas. It also comes in creams and lotion formulas. Vitamin C supplements can contain only rose hips or may include rose hips along with other sources of ascorbic acid. Powdered supplements are easy to take.

Complementary Agents: bioflavonoids, grape seed or pine bark proanthocyanidins, calcium/magnesium, capsicum, alfalfa, vitamin E

References

Dreher, F. and H. Maibach. 2001. Protective effects of topical antioxidants in humans. *Curr Probl Dermatol* 29:157–64.

Nutrition: Vitamin C. 2001. *Harvard Health Letter* Apr:26(6):4–5.

Sakuma et al. 2001. Ascorbic acid protects against peroxidative modification of low-density lipoprotein, maintaining its recognition by LDL receptors. *J Nutr Sci Vitaminol (Tokyo)* 47(1):28–31.

Smirnoff et al. 2001. Biosynthesis of ascorbic acid in plants: A Renaissance. *Annu Rev Plant Physiol Plant Mol Biol* 52:437–467.

Steenvoorden et al. 1999. Protection against UV-induced systemic immunosuppression in mice by a single topical application of the antioxidant vitamins C and E. *Int J Radiat Biol* 75(6):747–55.

Sarsaparilla *(Smilax ornata)*

Overview: Native to the Pacific coast of Mexico, sarsaparilla was used with sassafras to make root beer. Compounds found in this herb promote the production of testosterone and progesterone as well as cleansing the blood of toxins. This herb is routinely included in formulas designed to balance hormones. The sarsaparilla root contains a rich assortment of therapeutic compounds. Sarsparilla has a long history of use for female disorders and skin diseases (even leprosy).

Therapeutic Applications: blood disorders, male and female hormonal imbalances, infertility, menopausal symptoms, joint aches, gout, psoriasis, eczema, sexual dysfunction, skin problems, rheumatoid arthritis.

Scientific Updates: Clinical tests have discovered antibiotic attributes in sarsaparilla, due primarily to its saponin content. Sarsaparilla also has strong diuretic properties and dramatically lowers the urea content of the blood. Chinese research found that as a tonic, sarsaparilla can help rejuvenate the nerves, blood and glands. Sarsaparilla contains steroidal saponins, such as sarsasapogenin, which may imitate the action of some hormones. It also contains phytosterols, such as beta-sitosterol, which have documented pharmaceutical actions in the body. Other studies reveal its anti-inflammatory and hepato (liver) protective action. New data also points to its antivenom properties.

Safety: Sarsaparilla has been known to cause nausea and may even result in kidney damage if taken for long periods of time. Do not take this herb is pregnant or nursing or if taking digitalis or bismuth (the pink stuff). Breathing in sarsaparilla root particles can also cause asthma.

Special Instructions: To get optimal results, capsulized forms should be used; take between 5 to 9 grams of the capsulized dried root daily. Tinctures are commonly used at 3 ml doses taken three times daily.

Product Availability: Sarsaparilla is usually taken in combination with other natural compounds for maximum effect.

Complementary Agents: saw palmetto, licorice, damiana, ginseng, kelp, squaw vine, black cohosh, milk thistle, red raspberry, bee pollen, bee propolis, vitamin E, vitamin C, bioflavonoids, folic acid, calcium/magnesium, zinc, marine lipids, natural progesterone, soy isoflavones

References

Ageel et al. 1989. Experimental studies on antirheumatic crude drugs used in Saudi traditional medicine. *Drugs Exp Clin Res* 15:369–72.

Alam et al. 1994. Isolation, purification and partial characterization of viper venom inhibiting factor from the root extract of the Indian medicinal plant sarsaparilla (Hemidesmus indicus R. Br.). *Toxicon* 32(12):1551–7.

Duke, J.A. 1985. *CRC Handbook of Medicinal Herbs.* Boca Raton, FL: CRC Press. p. 446.

Rafatullah et al. 1991. Hepatoprotective and safety evaluation studies on sarsaparilla. *Int J Pharmacognosy* 29:296–301.

Vandenplas et al. 1996. Occupational asthma caused by sarsaparilla root dust. *J Allergy Clin Immunol* 97(6):1416–8.

Saw Palmetto *(Serenoa repens)*

Overview: The saw palmetto berry was used by ancient Mayans to treat disorders of the genitourinary tract and as an aphrodisiac. Interestingly, scientists today are discovering that compounds in saw palmetto can prevent the conversion of testosterone to dihydrotestosterone. This process helps to prevent the development of prostate disease. The herb is considered an overall glandular tonic. The sales of saw palmetto have dramatically increased as new studies confirm its positive action on the male urinary system and prostate gland.

Therapeutic Applications: prostate disease, genitourinary problems, endocrine disorders, infertility, impotence, bronchitis, colds, menstrual disorders, ovarian dysfunction, lactation, thyroid deficiencies, digestive problems, painful periods

Scientific Updates: Some studies suggest that saw palmetto may be a viable alternative to the use of Proscar, a pharmaceutical drug used for treating enlarged prostate glands. One three-year German study reported that a saw palmetto extract benefitted over 80 percent of men with mild to moderate BPH. In addition, this herb may exert anti-cancer effects on prostate tissue. Saw palmetto is also included in digestive formulas because of its ability to stimulate normal appetite and boost nutrient assimilation. Saw palmetto may also be useful for women who suffer from hormonal imbalances by helping to normalize estrogen levels.

Safety: Saw Palmetto is considered generally safe and very few side effects have been reported from its use. You may experience mild nausea and abdominal discomfort, but this is rare. If you have prostate disease, check with your physician before using saw palmetto or any other product.

Special Instructions: It is the sterol and fatty acid content of this herb that appears to benefit the prostate gland. Using it in conjunction with a diet that emphasizes cold-water fish, olive oil, and plenty of fresh fruits and vegetables can have a dramatic impact on the prostate gland.

Product Availability: Saw palmetto is available in capsules, softgels, liquids and standardized extracts. Teas are not as effective. Look for products that are standardized to an 85 to 95 percent fatty acids and sterol content. You may find it combined with pygeum *(Pygeum africanum)*, pumpkin seeds and essential fatty acids in prostate support formulas.

Complementary Agents: B-complex, calcium/magnesium, calcium carbonate, ginger, proanthocyanidins, phytonutrients, essential fatty acids, bee pollen, fennel, catnip, peppermint, capsicum, acidophilus, kelp, sarsaparilla, ginseng, pumpkin seeds, pygeum

References
Bach, D. and L. Ebeling. 1995. Long-term drug treatment of benign prostatic hyperpla-

sia: Results of a prospective three-year multicenter study using Sabal extract IDS 89. *Urologe* 35:178–83.

Gerber, G. 2000. Saw palmetto for the treatment of men with lower urinary tract symptoms. *J Urol* 163(5):1408–12.

Marks et al. 2001. Tissue effects of saw palmetto and finasteride: use of biopsy cores for in situ quantification of prostatic androgens. *Urology* 57(5):999–1005.

Marks et al. 2000. Effects of a saw palmetto herbal blend in men with symptomatic benign prostatic hyperplasia. *J Urol* 163(5):1451–6.

Paubert-Braquet et al. 1998. Effect of the lipidosterolic extract of Serenoa repens (Permixon) and its major components on basic fibroblast growth factor-induced proliferation of cultures of human prostate biopsies. *Eur Urol* 33(3):340–47.

Schizandra *(Schisandra chinensis)*

Overview: Schizandra is used an important tonic medicine by Chinese practitioners for fatigue and debility and to increase overall stamina. Schizandra comes from a tiny fruit that belongs to the magnolia family. Considered one of the best adaptogenic herbs for promoting well-being and vitality, it was used by people facing harsh physical demands. It has also been used to soften the skin, support the reproductive glands and sharpen the senses. Russian practitioners use it for diabetes, and its immunostimulant properties make it ideal for anyone with compromised immunity.

Therapeutic Applications: stress, weakness, fatigue, post surgery, immune malfunction, during chemotherapy, athletic endurance, chronic infections, diarrhea

Scientific Updates: Studies suggest that schizandra may enhance aerobic capacity and boost mental functions and mood. Another study was able to isolate a compound from schizandra that had anti-HIV properties. It has also shown liver-protective action even against toxic aflatoxins and appears to speed liver detoxification. It has also been linked with heart protection and improved endurance. It is the rich lignin content of this herb that is thought to account for its numerous medicinal actions. Lignins also stimulate the immune system.

Safety: The herb is considered safe; however, it may cause mild indigestion or rash. It should not be used by pregnant women as it may stimulate uterine contractions.

Special Instructions: Taking schizandra with herbs like ginseng for energy and with compounds like transfer factor for immune enhancement is recommended for optimal results.

Product Availability: Schizandra is available in capsules and liquid extracts and is commonly added to formulas designed to support the immune system or to provide added energy and stamina.

References

Azizov, A. and R. Seifulla. 1998. The effect of elton, leveton, fitoton and adapton on the work capacity of experimental animals. *Eksp Klin Farmakol* 61(3):61–63.

Bol'shakova et al. 1997. Antioxidant properties of a series of extracts from medicinal plants. *Biofizika* 42(2):480–3

Ip et al. 1996. Effect of a lignan-enriched extract of Schisandra chinensis on aflatoxin B1 and cadmium chloride-induced hepatotoxicity in rats. *Pharmacol Toxicol* 78(6):413–16.

Lee et al. 1999. Structure-activity relationships of lignans from Schisandra chinensis as platelet activating factor antagonists. *Biol Pharm Bull* 22(3):265–7.

Li et al. 1996. Schisandra chinensis-dependent myocardial protective action of sheng-mai-san in rats. *Am J Chin Med* 24(3–4):255–62.

Panossian et al. 1999. Effects of heavy physical exercise and adaptogens on nitric oxide content in human saliva. *Phytomedicine* 6(1):17–26.

Sun et al. 1996. Nigranoic acid, a triterpenoid from Schisandra sphaerandra that inhibits HIV-1 reverse transcriptase. *J Nat Prod* 59(5):525–27.

Zhu et al. 1999. Evaluation of the protective effects of Schisandra chinensis on Phase I drug metabolism using a CCl4 intoxication model. *J Ethnopharmacol* 67(1):61–8.

Skullcap *(Scutellaria lateriflora* and *S. baicalensis)*

Overview: Skullcap, named for its flower formation, acts as a sedative without the deleterious effects of narcotic drugs. It has a relaxing and sleep-promoting action which can help to quiet nervousness and treat insomnia. It has also been used in assisting with drug and alcohol withdrawal, for headaches, and as a natural muscle relaxant. It has also been used to treat anxiety, nervous tension and even menstrual cramps, epilepsy and drug withdrawal.

Therapeutic Applications: anxiety, insomnia, muscle spasms, neuralgia, tension, hysteria, pain, PMS, tension headaches, stress-related symptoms

Scientific Updates: Very few western studies have been done on this herb. Russian studies on a another skullcap species suggest that it may benefit stress-related symptoms and may even fight fungal and viral infections. In addition, anticancer compounds have also been identified in this herb and some studies suggest that it may potentiate chemotherapy treatments for cancer. It also has significant antioxidant properties and helps oxygenize brain tissue. The scutellarin content of skullcap may be responsible for its muscle relaxant and sedative actions.

Safety: Pregnant or nursing women should not use skullcap. Large doses may cause dizziness or lack of focus. It should not be combined with pharmaceutical hypnotics, alcohol or tranquilizers. In some studies, scullcap has been associated with potential liver damage although its combination with other herbs like mistletoe may explain the reaction.

Special Instructions: Taking any herbal sedative combination for insomnia works best if taken twenty minutes before retiring. While most people do not experience "morning hangover" effects, using melatonin with sedative herbs may result in a dulled feeling that can carry over into the day. While herbal sedatives are not considered habit forming, they should not be taken for indefinite periods of time.

Product Availability: Skullcap is available in liquid extracts, capsules and teas. You will often see it combined with herbs like valerian or passionflower in formulas designed to treat insomnia, headaches and nervous tension.

Complementary Agents: valerian root, chamomile, hops, passionflower, St.John's wort, wood betony, melatonin, B-complex, folic acid, calcium/magnesium

References

Bruseth, S. and A. Enge. 1992. Scullcap—liver damage; Mistletoe hepatitis. *Tidsskr Nor Laegeforen* 112(18):2389–90.

Gabrielska et al. 1997. Antioxidant activity of flavones from Scutellaria baicalensis in lecithin liposomes. *Z Naturforsch* 52(11–12):817–23.

Khazanov, V. and R. Saifutdinov. 1999. Mitochondrial mechanism of the anti-hypoxia effect of the Baikal scullcap extract . *Biull Eksp Biol Med* 128(9):327–9.

Razina et al. 2000. Medicinal plant preparations used as adjuvant therapeutics in experimental oncology. *Eksp Klin Farmakol* 63(5):59–61.

Razina et al. 1998. A semisynthetic flavonoid from the Baikal skullcap (Scutellaria baicalensis) as an agent to enhance the efficacy of chemotherapy in experimental tumors. *Eksp Klin Farmakol* 61(2):54–56.

Senna *(Cassia acutofolia)*

Overview: Senna is a powerful purgative herb that acts as an intestinal cleanser and strong laxative. It grows in shrub form in regions of the Nile. Today, it is commonly added to colonic formulas to stimulate peristalsis of the large intestine. Senna has traditionally been used to treat constipation and to purge or cleanse the bowels. Native Americans used it to treat fevers, hemorrhoids and parasite infection. Today, some over-the-counter laxative products use senna extracts.

Therapeutic Applications: constipation, jaundice, gallbladder disease, liver disease, worms

Scientific Updates: Anthraquinone compounds give senna its laxative effect and stimulate the bowels to move within six to eight hours of ingestion. These compounds do not work directly on the bowels, but are absorbed through the walls of the small intestine and subsequently stimulate the nerves of the large intestine. Some studies have found that senna was comparable to a laxative drug called lactulose. Other studies suggest that it has the ability to relieve pain, calm the central nervous system and has antimicrobial actions.

Safety: Because senna is absorbed systemically, it should not be used by pregnant or nursing mothers. Anyone with colon diseases should not use this herb unless it is part of a carefully designed formula. Taking senna can cause significant gripping pains in the abdomen, suggesting that it should always be taken as part of a combination. Senna can become habit forming if taken in excess or for long periods of time. Other potential side effects include: diarrhea, nausea and abdominal cramps. If any of these occur, discontinue use. People with intestinal diseases and those taking licorice, thiazide, corticosteroids or diuretics should not take senna. It is not for children. Extended use or abuse can also cause potassium loss and dehydration, which could affect the heart. California requires warning labels for products that contain senna. Senna can also decrease the absorption of certain drugs.

Special Instructions: It's best not to take senna as a single supplement. Combining it with ginger and other laxative herbs helps to prevent abdominal cramping. There are several herbs such as cascara sagrada, which are milder and are not considered habit forming.

Product Availability: Senna is available in capsules, teas and liquid extracts. It is commonly added to laxative formulas.

Complementary Agents: aloe vera, ginger, peppermint, fennel, cascara sagrada, slippery elm, black walnut, calcium/magnesium, essential fatty acids, marine lipids, digestive enzymes, acidophilus, cloves

References

Agra et al. 1998. Efficacy of senna versus lactulose in terminal cancer patients treated with opioids. *Jour Pain Symptom Manage* 15(1):1–7.

Ali et al. 1997. Some effects of Cassia italica on the central nervous system in mice. *J Pharm Pharmacol* 49(5):500–04.

Fugh-Berman, A. 2000. Herb-drug interactions. *Lancet* 8:355(9198):134–8.

Mukhopadhyay et al. 1998. Genotoxicity of sennosides on the bone marrow cells of mice. *Food Chem Toxicol* 36(11):937–40.

Sansores-Peraza et al. 2000. An antimicrobial alkaloid from Senna racemosa. *Fitoterapia* 71(6):690–2.

Slippery Elm *(Ulmus fulva)*

Overview: Slippery elm is a mucilaginous compound that comes from elm tree bark. It was used for generations by Native Americans to soothe irritated mucous membranes. Its protective and healing action make it an excellent herb for treating diarrhea, colon disorders, sore throats or intestinal ulcers. Ancient practitioners mixed the powdered herb with water creating a "slurry" for use on burns and other skin injuries or inflammations and even consumed it as a food. It later became widely used for coughs and colds. It was also recommended for diarrhea, ulcers and heartburn.

Therapeutic Applications: abscesses, asthma, bronchitis, Crohn's disease, colitis, constipation, coughs, diarrhea, digestive disorders, lung ailments, gastritis, ulcers, heartburn, sore throats. Topical applications: burns, rashes and minor wounds

Scientific Updates: Although there is a lack of scientific study on this herb, its high mucilage content has proven its value for the treatment of diarrhea, coughs, stomach upsets, colitis and a variety of lung problems. The antitussive action of slippery elm can soothe raw throats and inhibit chronic coughing. In addition, the high mucilage content of this herb helps to heal and restore the mucous membranes of the GI tract. Studies on related elm species support its medicinal uses. The fact that slippery elm is found in over-the-counter medications in the United States and Britain attests to its versatility. Slippery elm is commonly found in lozenges and in topical form can promote skin healing and soothe rashes. The high mucilage content of this herb is responsible for its protective and healing properties.

Safety: This herb has no known toxicity. It has been used as a food and is considered safe for children.

Special Instructions: Open capsules of slippery elm powder and mix them into applesauce or other soft foods; give such a mixture to babies and small children for diarrhea. Adults should take up to 5 grams of the powder mixed with water prior to meals.

Product Availability: Slippery elm is available as a dried powder, capsules, lozenges, liquid extracts, and as a tea. It is often added in formulas designed to treat colds, flu, sore throats, diarrhea and urinary tract infections.

Complementary Agents: marshmallow, fenugreek, saw palmetto, mullein, thyme, pumpkin seed, yucca, aloe vera, capsicum, horehound, yerba santa, wild cherry, vitamin C, bioflavonoids, vitamin A, B-complex, vitamin E, zinc, acidophilus

References

Jun et al. 1998. Inhibition of nitric oxide synthesis by butanol fraction of the methanol extract of Ulmus davidiana in murine macrophages. *J Ethnopharmacol* 62(2):129–35.

Kim et al. 1996. Sesquiterpene O-naphthoquinones from the root bark of Ulmus davidiana. *Phytochemistry* 43(2):425–30.

Ody, Penelope. 1993. *The Complete Medicinal Herbal* Dorling-Kindersley, New York. p. 152.

Squaw Vine (Mitchella repens)

Overview: Squaw vine (also known as partridge berry) was extensively used by Native Americans as a pregnancy tonic. It was believed to strengthen uterine contractions and ease childbirth. Today it is used in female corrective formulas dealing with menstrual disorders.

Therapeutic Applications: childbirth, menstrual disorders, miscarriage, skin problems, female tonic, uterine disorders, vaginal yeast infections

Scientific Updates: There are few studies on the herb. Traditional herbalists use it in herbal combinations designed to correct female complaints or strengthen the female reproductive system. Some herbalists believe it acts as an effective diuretic as well. Its traditional use has been as a uterine tonic and stimulant to the ovaries.

Safety: Use as directed in appropriate doses. If pregnant or nursing, check with your physician before using squaw vine.

Special Instructions: I recommend taking squaw vine in tea form. You can combine it with red raspberry for synergistic action.

Product Availability: Squaw vine can be purchased as a tea, in capsule form or as a liquid extract.

Complementary Agents: kelp, red raspberry, wild yam, black cohosh, dong quai, damiana, cramp bark, licorice, queen of the meadow, saw palmetto, vitamin E, vitamin C, bioflavonoids, folic acid

References

Ody, Penelope. 1993. *The Complete Medicinal Herbal* Dorling-Kindersley, New York. p. 152.

Ritchason, Jack. 1994. *The Little Herb Encyclopedia.* Pleasant Grove, Utah: Woodland Publishing.

St. John's Wort *(Hypericum perforatum)*

Overview: Used for wound healing during the Crusades, St. John's wort has the ability to cleanse tissue and reduce inflammation. Its ability to act as a natural antidepressant has recently made it one of the most sought after herbs in modern history. Recent European studies have confirmed its application for depression and anxiety. It also has impressive antiviral properties and when used in topical form can promote healing, while inhibiting infection and inflammation. It contains a very active compound called hypericum, which is believed to give it a wide array of therapeutic applications.

Therapeutic Applications: AIDS, after-birth pains, cancer, menstrual cramps, mild depression, viral infections, bacterial infections, sleep disorders, wounds and burns, nicotene withdrawal, weight loss, PMS, Parkinson's disease, arthritis

Scientific Updates: In 1942, a compound called hypericin was isolated from the St. John's wort plant and used as a natural antidepressant. The National Institutes of Health (NIH) has intitated the first U.S. clinical trial of St. John's wort. Other studies have concluded that St. John's wort is more effective than placebo in treating mild to moderate depression and that it compares to some prescription antidepressants with less side effects. Its antiviral and antifungal properties have also been investigated and confirmed, especially for AIDS. For depression, it is thought to increase serotonin levels, although its exact mechanism remains unknown. It may also help with nicotine withdrawal. PMS and with weight loss.

Safety: Some experts believe this herb can cause severe photosensitivity (light sensitivity), although incidence is rare in humans—with the exception of AIDS patients who have taken large doses. One recent study disputes this effect. Exposure to strong sunlight for anyone with fair skin, however, is not recommended. Because St. John's wort may be an MAO inhibitor, tyramine containing foods (cheeses, beer, wine, herring, yeast, etc.) should be avoided when taking the herb. Do not take St. John's wort with L-dopa or any protease inhibitors. Pregnant or nursing women should avoid St. John's wort. Do not take it if undergoing general anesthesia; never stop taking any drug without the approval and supervision of your physician. Take this herb with food to avoid stomach upset. If taken too close to bedtime, St. John's wort may cause insomnia.

Drugs that St. John's Wort May Affect:

AIDS/HIV antiviral medications including:
- protease inhibitors such as indinavir, nelfinavir, and ritonavir, and non-nucleoside reverse transcriptase inhibitors (NNRTIs)
- oral contraceptives
- warfarin (a blood thinner) and digoxin
- epilepsy drugs such as phenytoin
- asthma medications,such as theophylline
- immune modulaters such as cyclosporin

Special Instructions: For topical applications, use St. John's wort oil three times daily on affected areas. Decoctions or tea soaked cotton cloths can be used as compresses. For depression, take 300 mg of a 0.3 percent hypericin product three times daily. If you have AIDS, be aware that this herb should not be taken with protease inhibitors.

Product Availability: Look for supplements with a standardized 0.3 percent hypericin content. St. John's wort is available in capsules, tinctures, teas and in bulk products. Taking it with B-vitamins is recommended.

Complementary Agents: vitamin B-complex, folic acid, calcium/magnesium, essential fatty acids, ginkgo, tyrosine, essential fatty acids

References

Greeson et al. 2001. St. John's wort (Hypericum perforatum): a review of the current pharmacological, toxicological, and clinical literature. *Psychopharmacology (Berl)* 153(4):402–14.

James, J. 2000. St. John's wort warning: do not combine with protease inhibitors, NNRTIs. *AIDS Treat News* 18:337:3–5.

Linde et al. 1996. St John's Wort for Depression-an Overview and Meta-Analysis of Randomized Clinical Trials. *British Medical Journal* 313(7052):253–258.

Perovic et al. 1995. Pharmacological Profile of Hypericum Extract. Effect on Serotonin Uptake by Postsynaptic Receptors. *Arzneimittelforschung* 45(11):1145–1148.

Schempp et al. 2001. Single-dose and steady-state administration of Hypericum perforatum extract (St John's Wort) does not influence skin sensitivity to UV radiation, visible light, and solar-simulated radiation. *Arch Dermatol* 137(4):512–3.

Shelton et al. 2001. Effectiveness of St John's wort in major depression: a randomized controlled trial. *JAMA* 18:285:1978–86.

Upton et al. 1997. St. John's Wort (Hypericum perforatum): Quality Control, Analytical and Therapeutic Monograph. Santa Cruz, CA. *American Herbal Pharmacopoeia.* p. 4.

Thyme *(Thymus vulgaris)*

Overview: Used by the ancient Greeks for its aromatic properties, thyme works to relax stomach spasms and promotes healing. Thymol, or thyme oil, is used in Listerine for its antiseptic action. Thyme, a member of the mint family, is famous for its ability to season meat and fish. Egyptians used thyme for embalming. Many have used it for headaches, digestive upsets, and respiratory disorders and infections. Its antiseptic action made it popular for topical applications, and many use its aromatic properties to elevate mood.

Therapeutic Applications: bronchitis, coughs, digestive ailments, gas, gingivitis, gout, headaches, laryngitis, lung disorders, sciatica, sore throat, stomach problems, throat maladies, worms, pertussis (whooping cough), headaches, gastric ulcers, urinary infections and menstrual cramps, mouth sores, gum disease, hair loss

Scientific Updates: The thymol content of thyme works as an expectorant and cough suppressant. It is frequently used in cough syrups prescribed for lung ailments like bronchitis. When combined with fenugreek and thyme, it may relive the pain of migraine headaches. The carminative properties of thyme make it an effective treatment for stomach upsets. One study found that thyme oil scalp massage benefitted some people with hair loss. It acts against bacteria like *E. coli* and fungi like candida, and it has significant antioxidant actions. It has also shown activity against the *H. pylori* bacteria associated with the formation of gastric ulcers.

Safety: As is the case with most herbs, the essential oil form of thyme is much more powerful and should not be used internally. Pregnant women should avoid thyme. Excessive doses may stimulate uterine contractions. It should not be used by anyone with a thyroid disorder. Direct contact with thyme dust can cause dermatitis in certain individuals.

Special Instructions: The essential oil form of thyme can be used in massage or aromatherapy dispensers for mental stress, PMS, fatigue and melancholia. In addition, thyme oil has natural antiseptic actions. You can add thyme oil to other carriers and apply it to minor skin injuries. Rub thyme oil on the temples to relieve a headache.

Product Availability: Thyme is available as a whole herb, an essential oil, in liquid extracts and in capsules. It is often added in formulas designed to treat colds, flu, respiratory infections and headaches.

Complementary Agents: fenugreek, feverfew, capsicum, yerba santa, marshmallow, mullein, saw palmetto, wild cherry, licorice, vitamin C, bioflavonoids, vitamin A, acidophilus

References
Haraguchi et al. 1996. Antiperoxidative components in Thymus vulgaris. *Planta Medica* 62(3):217–21.

Hay et al. 1998. Randomized trial of aromatherapy. Successful treatment for alopecia areata. *Arch Dermatol* 134(11):1349–52.

Inouye et al. 2001. Antibacterial activity of essential oils and their major constituents against respiratory tract pathogens by gaseous contact. *J Antimicrob Chemother* 47(5):565–73.

Kulevanova et al. 2000. Investigation of antimicrobial activity of essential oils of several Macedonian Thymus L. species (Lamiaceae). *Boll Chim Farm* 139(6):276–80.

Spiewak et al. 2001. Occupational airborne contact dermatitis caused by thyme dust. *Contact Dermatitis* 44(4):235–9.

Tabak et al. 1996. In vitro inhibition of Helicobacter pylori by extracts of thyme. *J Appl Bacteriol* 80(6):667–72.

Takacsova et al. 1995. Study of the antioxidative effects of thyme, sage, juniper and oregano. *Nahrung* 39(3):241–3.

Uva Ursi *(Arctostaphylos uva-ursi)*

Overview: Also known as bearberry, the leaves and berries of this sturdy plant have been used to treat urinary tract infections. Apart from being smoked like tobacco in some cultures, it was also utilized for weight-loss and for kidney disorders. Because it contains a compound called arbutin, uva ursi has the ability to drain excess water from cells. This promotes an antiseptic effect on the kidneys and reduces acidity while acting as a natural diuretic.

Therapeutic Applications: bladder infections, Bright's disease, cystitis, diabetes, nephritis, pyelo-nephritis, water retention, liver ailments, chronic diarrhea

Scientific Updates: The primary constituent of uva ursi is the glycoside arbutin, which is responsible for the herb's diuretic action. In addition, when it is excreted from the kidneys, arbutin produces an antiseptic effect on the mucous membranes of the urinary tract. Chemical compounds in uva ursi also help to balance the pH of urine. American research has found that uva ursi is effective against nephritis and kidney stones and possesses all-around tonic properties. The hydroquinone content of uva ursi has potent antimicrobial properties, especially in the urine and may also potentiate the action of cortisone drugs.

Safety: Gastric irritation and nausea can occur with this herb and experts advise against its long-term use. Don't take acid producing compounds like vitamin C or citrus fruit juices with uva ursi, since it works best when the urine is alkaline. Neither pregnant women nor children should use uva ursi. Do not take it for more than two weeks.

Special Instructions: Look for products with a standardized content of 20 percent arbutin. Tinctures are usually taken in 5 ml doses three times daily. Capsule dosages vary from 250 to 500 mg three times daily. Do not use uva ursi to treat a urinary tract infection without consulting your physician.

Product Availability: Uva ursi is available as a single herb but is more commonly taken in combinations designed to treat urinary tract infections that include juniper berries, buchu and cranberry.

Complementary Agents: parsley, buchu, alfalfa, cornsilk, juniper berries, marshmallow, cranberry, lemon grass, proanthocyanidins, mineral and electrolyte supplements

References

Jahodar et al. 1985. Antimicrobial effect of arbutin and an extract of the leaves of Arctostaphylos uva-ursi in vitro. *Ceskoslov Farm* 34:174–8.

Matsuda et al. 1992. Pharmacological studies on leaf of Arctostaphylos uva-ursi (L) Spreng. V. Effect of water extract from Arctostaphylos uva-ursi (L) Spreng (bearberry leaf) on the antiallergic and anti-inflammatory activities of dexamethasone ointment. *J Pharm Soc Japan* 112:673–7.

Valerian Root *(Valeriana officinalis)*

Overview: Valerian root grows in temperate areas and was brought to America by early settlers. Valerian has accrued some impressive credentials as a well-respected treatment for insomnia, emotional upset, and anxiety without the risk of addiction or serious side effects. It was also used by ancient Greek practitioners for digestive ailments and epilepsy. The ester-containing compounds in this herb give it a characteristic odor and promote its safe and natural sedating effect.

Therapeutic Applications: insomnia, headaches, panic attacks, hyperexcitability, hypertension, heart disorders, afterbirth pains, anxiety, tension, high blood pressure, stress, nervous stomach, palpitations, menstrual cramps, muscle spasms, irritable bowel, altitude sickness

Scientific Updates: Valerian tranquilizes and regulates the autonomic nervous system, enhances higher brain functions, and eases childhood psychosomatic disturbances and behavioral disorders. Valerian seems to improve sleep quality with none of the drawbacks of barbiturates. It is also recommended for anyone who suffers from cardiovascular disease or hypertension in that it helps to relax smooth muscle and ease tension. One study recently confirmed that taking hops and valerian together was as effective as benzodiazepines (Valium and Xanax) for test subjects with simple insomnia. It is now thought that valerian root actually affects serotonin and gamma aminobutyric acid (GABA), which are involved in the process of relaxation and sleep.

Safety: Valerian has low toxicity. Pregnant or nursing women and children under the age of twelve should not use valerian. It should never be combined with other sedatives or with alcohol and should not be taken prior to activities requiring full mental focus. If taken for extended periods of time, valerian may cause headaches and restlessness. Some people experience the paradox effect in which valerian actually stimulates them. An upset stomach may also occur after taking valerian. Its safety for people with kidney or liver disease has not been determined. Do not exceed recommended doses. If you are taking drugs for insomnia or anxiety, do not take valerian.

Special Instructions: For insomnia, the standard dose of valerian is 270 to 450 mg of a valerian extract, taken thirty minutes before retiring. A reduced dose may work for anxiety.

Product Availability: Valerian can be purchased in capsules, caplets, liquid extracts, teas, and in timed-released supplements. You will often see valerian combined with other nervine or sedative herbs such as kava and in formulas designed to treat anxiety, insomnia and menstrual disorders. European manufacturers now offer odorless valerian products, which are not yet available in this country.

Complementary Agents: hops, chamomile, passionflower, kava, skullcap, licorice, mullein, marshmallow, wood betony, hawthorn berries, black cohosh, niacin, calcium/magnesium, vitamin B6, melatonin

References

Giedke, H. and U. 2000. Breyer-Pfaff. Critical evaluation of the effect of valerian extract on sleep structure and sleep quality. *Pharmacopsychiatry* 33(6):239.

Lindahl, O. and L. Lindwall. 1989. Double-blind study of a valerian preparation. *Pharmacology Biochemistry and Behavior* 32(4):1065–66.

Stevinson, C. and E. Ernst. 2000. Valerian for insomnia: a systematic review of random-ized clinical trials. *Sleep Med* 1:1(2):91–99.

Volz, H. 2001. Phytochemicals as means to induce sleep. *Arztl Fortbild Qualitatssich* 95(1):33–4.

Vonderheid-Guth et al. 2000. Pharmacodynamic effects of valerian and hops extract combination (Ze 91019) on the quantitative-topographical EEG in healthy volunteers. *Eur J Med Res* 19:5(4):139–44.

Wagner et al. 1998. Beyond benzodiazepines: alternative pharmacologic agents for the treatment of insomnia. *Ann Pharmacother* 32(6):680–91.

White Willow *(Salix alba)*

Overview: As one of the first herbs to interest scientists, the white willow tree grows in areas scattered all over the world. It is most famous for its natural content of acetylsalicylic acid from which aspirin was derived. In fact, it provided the natural basis for the manufacture of aspirin decades ago. While it is less potent than synthetic aspirin applications, it also comes with fewer side effects.

Therapeutic Applications: pain, bursitis, fever, headache, osteoarthritis, rheumatoid arthritis, muscle strains, sprains, menstrual cramps

Scientific Updates: A compound called glycoside salicin found in white willow gives the herb its natural anti-inflammatory and analgesic properties. As a pain reliever, it takes longer to act; but its effects may actually have more longevity than conventional aspirin preparations. In one study, the use of willow bark for back pain showed that it did provide significant relief with no stomach problems. In another trial, the same type of effects were noted in people suffering from osteoarthritis. White willow bark is rich in compounds called tannins, which have medicinal effects in the stomach and intestinal tract.

Safety: Do not use white willow for extended periods of time or stomach upset or the development of ulcers is possible. Like aspirin, do not give to children with any viral infections. If you are already taking aspirin therapy, NSAIDs or blood thinners, check with your doctor before taking white willow. It is not advised for pregnant or nursing women, people with allergies to aspirin, ulcers, bleeding disorders or diabetes. Do not use white willow if you are phenytoin or valproate. Always check with your doctor if you are on any drug before taking white willow.

Special Instructions: White willow can be made into a tea by placing 1 gram of the bark in boiling water for ten minutes. Three to five cups can be taken daily. In tincture form, it is commonly taken in 1 to 2 ml doses three times daily. Historical or traditional use: white willow's Latin name is the source of the name for acetylsalicylic acid (aspirin), as well as the parent compound from which aspirin was eventually created. If you are taking a standardized product, the daily dose of salicin should range from 60 to 120 mg daily.

Product Availability: White willow can be purchased as a tea, in capsules, extracts or in supplements that have standardized salicin content. This herb is often added to formulas designed to treat fevers and joint pain. Fluid extracts are stronger than tinctures.

Complementary Agents: elderberry, boneset, gentian, marshmallow, plantain

References

Chrubasik et al. 2000. Treatment of low back pain exacerbations with willow bark extract: a randomized double-blind study. *Am J Med* 109:9–14.

Meier et al. 1988. Pharmaceutical aspects of the use of willows in herbal remedies. *Planta Med* 54:559–560.

Ody, Penelope. 1993. *The Complete Medicinal Herbal.* New York: Dorling-Kindersley. p. 94

Schmid et al. 1998. Efficacy and tolerability of a standardized willow bark extract in patients with osteoarthritis: randomized, placebo-controlled, double-blind clinical trial. *FACT* 3:186.

Wild Cherry *(Prunus virginiana or serotina)*

Overview: Wild cherry can help calm dry coughs and lubricate irritated mucous membranes. It was used in old-fashioned lozenges because of its cough soothing properties.

Therapeutic Applications: allergies, asthma, congestion, coughs, colds, sore throats, bronchitis, fever, tuberculosis

Scientific Updates: While there are few clinical studies on this herb, wild cherry is believed to soothe irritated mucosal tissue and treat symptoms of respiratory distress. Herbal practitioners also believe that it can benefit asthmatics by relaxing the nerves that feed the lungs.

Safety: Wild cherry is generally regarded as safe if used in appropriate dosages. It does contain small amounts of cyanide, so you should not take it for extended periods of time or in large doses. Young children, pregnant or nursing women, or people with liver or kidney disease should not take wild cherry.

Special Instructions: Using wild cherry in liquid or lozenge form is recommended for coughs and sore throats.

Product Availability: Wild cherry is often added to cough syrups, cold preparations and lozenges. It is also available as a single supplement in tea, capsule or liquid form.

Complementary Agents: slippery elm, capsicum, fenugreek, yerba santa, mullein, saw palmetto, marshmallow, horehound, thyme, vitamin C, bioflavonoids, proanthocyanidins, noni, vitamin A, B-complex, vitamin B12, potassium, calcium/magnesium

References

Mowrey, Daniel Ph.D. 1986. *The Scientific Validation of Herbal Medicine.* Connecticut: Keats Publishing. p. 2.

Wild Yam, Mexican *(Dioscorea villosa)*

Overview: Traditionally used for its hormonal properties, wild yam root (also known as Mexican wild yam) is considered a phytoestrogen (progesterone), or precursor to progesterone. Wild yam comes from a large root that belongs to a vine that grows in this hemisphere. The Mexican variety of wild yam contains a saponin called diosgenin, which can be used to commercially manufacture progesterone. Diosgenin has become quite well known and is used in synthetic hormone products such as progesterone creams for the treatment of osteoporosis, menstrual disorders and menopause. While the herb contains phytoestrogenic compounds, it is not readily converted to progesterone in the body.

Therapeutic Applications: hormonal imbalance, PMS, menstrual disorders, infertility, mood swings, fibrocystic breasts, uterine fibroids, ovarian cysts, menopause, osteoporosis, cancer (hormonally related), fibromyalgia, prostate disease

Scientific Updates: Dr. John Lee's studies impressively delineate the ability of transdermal natural progesterone to effectively raise progesterone levels and balance out female hormone levels. Wild yam alone is not considered a true source of natural progesterone. Wild yam may help to prevent and treat certain cancers, as well as a myriad of hormonally-related symptoms. It also has proven antioxidant activity and appears to raise good cholesterol levels while reducing blood fats. It may also be of value for hard to treat diseases like fibromyalgia and chronic fatigue syndrome.

Safety: Considered safe and nontoxic if used in appropriate amounts. A contraceptive effect only occurs with extremely large doses.

Special Instructions: Topical applications of wild yam with added progesterone may help with PMS and menopausal symptoms. Look for products with guaranteed progesterone content.

Product Availability: Wild yam is available in capsules but is more often added to women's topical products, which combine it with progesterone designed to treat hormonal problems, menopause, and joint disorders.

Complementary Agents: dong quai, black cohosh, damiana, saw palmetto, sarsaparilla, soy isoflavones, vitamin E, vitamin B-complex, folic acid, essential fatty acids, vitamin C, bioflavonoids, grape seed/pine bark proanthocyanidins

References

Araghiniknam et al. 1996. Antioxidant activity of dioscorea and dehydroepiandrosterone (DHEA) in older humans. *Life Sci* 59(11):147–57.

Dykman et al. 1998. The effects of nutritional supplements on the symptoms of fibromyalgia and chronic fatigue syndrome. *Integr Physiol Behav Sci* 33(1):61–71.

Lee, John M.D. 1993. *What Your Doctor May Not Tell You About Menopause.*

Lee, John M.D. 1993. *Natural Progesterone: The Multiple Roles of a Remarkable Hormone.* Sebastopol, California: BLL Pub.

Wood Betony *(Betonica officinalis)*

Overview: Wood betony was used as a medieval remedy for head ailments. It grows readily in the hedges and meadows of Britain. It is the aerial parts of the plant that are used medicinally and were originally dried in the sun. Today it is used similarly as a nervine or calming herb. Its glycoside content appears to alleviate head pain and dilate blood vessels.

Therapeutic Applications: nervous disorders, headaches (especially tension), insomnia, hysteria, facial pain, migraines, liver protectant, Parkinson's disease, neuralgia

Scientific Updates: It is believed that wood betony has the ability to dilate blood vessels and promote relaxation. Its vascular effect has been linked to its ability to relieve headache pain, hence causing muscles to relax. It also appears to support the nervous system making it good for disorders related to anxiety or tension. It has also been used for certain types of neuralgia.

Safety: Wood betony is considered safe when taken in appropriate doses. Because it has the ability to mildly stimulate the uterus, it should be avoided in pregnancy.

Special Instructions: Wood betony tea can be made by pouring a cup of boiling water on 1 to 2 teaspoonfuls of the dried herb and steeping for fifteen minutes. Tea can be taken three times daily. Common tincture doses are 2 to 6 ml three times daily.

Product Availability: Wood betony can be purchased as a tea, in capsules or liquid extracts.

Complementary Agents: valerian, hops, skullcap, kava, marshmallow, mullein, chamomile, black cohosh, melatonin, lavender, vitamin B-complex, and calcium/magnesium

References

Mowrey, Daniel. 1986. *The Scientific Validation of Herbs.* New Canaan, Connecticut: Keats Publishing. p. 193.

Zinchenko, T. and I. Fefer. 1962. Investigation of glycosides from betonica officinalis. *Farmatsevt, Zhurnal* 17(3):35–38.

Yellow Dock *(Rumex crispus)*

Overview: As one of the best blood-cleansing herbs, yellow dock helps to rid the body of toxins and purges the lymph glands. It is unusually rich in iron and is an excellent liver tonic. As a member of the buckwheat family, its orange roots contain the majority of its therapeutic compounds. Used anciently for skin disorders and indigestion, it was considered a liver tonic and often added to dandelion preparations. As a "bitter" herb it has also been used to treat wounds and hemorrhoids, anemia, joint disorders and to stimulate the appetite.

Therapeutic Applications: acne, anemia, blood disorders, blood cleanser, boils, cancer, coughs, hives, iron deficiency, psoriasis, eczema, constipation, flatulence, liver ailments, rheumatism, skin disorders, sores, indigestion, sinusitis, respiratory infections

Scientific Updates: Traditional herbalists believe that yellow dock enhances the liver's ability to filter the blood and has antibacterial properties. It is considered one of the best herbal medications for skin problems. Some studies have succeeded at isolating certain compounds from this herb that show the ability to inhibit inflammatory agents in the body as well as antiviral properties. The herb is quite bitter due to its tannin content and is unusually rich in iron.

Safety: Yellow dock should be avoided during pregnancy and while breast feeding. In some people, it causes mild diarrhea or nausea. Do not eat fresh yellow dock leaves as they can be toxic. In certain sensitive individuals, yellow dock may cause an allergic reaction.

Special Instructions: Taking yellow dock as a part of a cleansing formula is recommended.

Product Availability: Yellow dock root is available as a liquid extract, in capsules, and as teas. You will commonly find it in formulas designed to support the skin and in detoxifying blends. It is also often added to dandelion and milk thistle for added effect.

Complementary Agents: dandelion, capsicum, burdock, garlic, milk thistle, fenugreek, quassia, kelp, black cohosh, red sage, red clover, noni, blue-green algae, vitamin C, vitamin A, bioflavonoids, B-complex, proanthocyanidins

References

Jager et al. 1996. Screening of Zulu medicinal plants for prostaglandin-synthesis inhibitors. *J Ethnopharmacol* 52(2):100.

Kang et al. 1996. Isolation and identification of two anthraquinones from Rumex gmelini. *Turcz Chung Kuo Chung Yao Tsa Chih* 21(12):741–42, 762.

Taylor et al. 1996. Antiviral activities of medicinal plants of southern Nepal. *J Ethnopharmacol* 53(2):97–104.

Yerba Maté

Overview: Also known as Paraguayan tea, this plant was considered a lung tonic to open respiratory passages. It also stimulates the productions of natural cortisone. For a time, maté (mah-tay) was used as a beverage until coffee became more popular. Maté tea made from the leaves and twigs is still used in South America for fatigue and to inhibit hunger, and is usually served in a traditional bulb-like pipe cup. Today the tea is used for its mildly stimulating properties and to enhance mental performance and alertness. It has also been used to increase stamina during times of physical stress and for weight loss.

Therapeutic Applications: allergies, asthma, bronchial congestion, cardiovascular disease, colds, flu, laryngitis, hemorrhoids, bladder infections, kidney and bladder stones, constipation, indigestion, hunger control

Scientific Updates: Recent findings suggest that water extracts of maté were more powerful than vitamin C for their antioxidant actions especially in reducing the dangerous oxidation of fats. It is the polyphenols found in maté that provide its strong antioxidant activity. Maté leaves are rich in calcium, magnesium, and potassium and may work to actually relax or dilate blood vessels, which benefits the heart and circulatory system. Maté also contains caffeine, theobromine and theophylline, all of which are stimulant compounds called xanthines. It contains less caffeine than coffee does ounce per ounce. Its ability to relax smooth muscle helps to explain its traditional use for respiratory diseases like asthma, and herbalists believe it enhances the action of other herbs.

Safety: Prolonged use or large doses of maté may cause nervousness, anxiety, nausea and dehydration. There has been a link drinking maté and an increased risk of esophageal and kidney cancer. Do not combine maté with other stimulants like caffeine or with alcohol. It is not for children, nor for pregnant or nursing women. If you are taking asthma drugs containing theophylline, do not use this herb. If you have any condition, check with your doctor before using maté.

Special Instructions: Tea forms of this herb are popular but must be chosen carefully to ensure purity and the absence of contaminants.

Product Availability: Maté is sold as a tea and a liquid extracts including mists. It is commonly found in blends designed to boost energy.

Complementary Agents: fenugreek, capsicum, mullein, marshmallow, slippery elm, wild cherry, comfrey, vitamin C, bioflavonoids, vitamin A, calcium/magnesium, green tea, proanthocyanidins

References

Gugliucci, A. 1996. Antioxidant effects of Ilex paraguariensis: induction of decreased oxidability of human LDL in vivo. *Biochem Biophys Res Commun* 224(2):338–44.

Gugliucci, A. and A. Stahl. 1995. Low density lipoprotein oxidation is inhibited by extracts of Ilex paraguariensis. *Biochem Mol Biol Int* 35(1):47–56.

Muccillo Baisch et al. 1998. Endothelium-dependent vasorelaxing activity of aqueous extracts of Ilex paraguariensis on mesenteric arterial bed of rats. *J Ethnopharmacol* 60(2):133–39.

Vasques, A. and P. Moyna. 1986. Studies on maté drinking. *Journal of Ethnopharmacology* 18(3):267–72.

Yucca *(Yucca schidigera and other species)*

Overview: Familiar to desert dwellers, this tree grows in dry arid climates. Historically, Native Americans used the slick and foamy liquid found in its leaves for various skin injuries and disorders. It was also used to reduce the inflammation seen in joint diseases and in muscle strains and sprains. Like the aloe plant, yucca leaves are rich in saponins, which have also been used in poultices and even in compresses for hair loss. Today, yucca is commonly recommended for arthritic conditions.

Therapeutic Applications: joint diseases (rheumatoid and osteoarthritis) muscle soreness, skin disorders (topically)

Scientific Updates: Yucca saponins give this plant its therapeutic value. Much like soap, they can dissolve in both fats and in water. One study suggested the possibility that yucca saponins block the release of certain toxic agents from the colon, which interfere with the formation of cartilage in the joints. Although this is only a theory, this blockage of toxic agents may explain yucca's use for arthritis. It also has anticancer properties and may help fight parasites like giardia.

Safety: Too much yucca tea can cause diarrhea. Because yucca is approved for use in foods that have foam (like root beer) scientists assume that the supplement is safe, although studies in pregnant or nursing mothers have not been conducted.

Special Instructions: Take capsules according to label instructions. For arthritis treatment, you may require larger doses. Yucca root tea can be made by boiling 1/4 ounce of the root in 2 cups of water for fifteen to twenty minutes. Yucca tea can be taken at 3 to 5 cups daily.

Product Availability: Yucca comes in capsules, water and alcohol based extracts and as a tea. It is commonly added to joint formulas.

Complementary Agents: glucosamine and chondroitin, MSM, malic acid, aloe vera, noni, grapeseed or pinebark extracts, calcium/magnesium

References

Bingham et al. 1975. Yucca plant saponin in the management of arthritis. *J Appl Nutr* 27:45–50.

McAllister et al. 2001. Studies on the use of Yucca schidigera to control giardiosis. *Vet Parasitol* 22:97(2):85–99.

Individual Vitamin Profiles

Two categories of vitamins exist: fat soluble and water soluble. We need to continually replenish water-soluble vitamins because they are routinely excreted and cannot be stored in the body. These include vitamin C and the B-complex vitamins. Although lipid or fat-based vitamins can accumulate in liver and fatty tissue, they still need to be continually replaced. These fat-based vitamins include vitamin A, D, E and K.

Fat-Soluble Vitamins

Vitamin A

Overview: Vitamin A is a fat-soluble micronutrient that is essential for vision, reproduction, immunity, tissue repair, and many other biological functions. Preformed vitamin A is obtained only from animal sources. Common supplemental forms include retinol and retinyl palmitate. Plant-derived carotenoids such as beta-carotene are converted to vitamin A in the body.

Daily Value: 5,000 international units (IU), or 1,500 retinol equivalents

Optimal Consumption: Average adult: 5,000 to 10,000 IU of preformed vitamin A. **Note:** You may add an additional 25,000 to 50,000 IU (15 to 30 mg) of beta-carotene or beta-carotene combined with mixed carotenoids.

Applications: acne, night blindness, macular degeneration, immune weakness, skin disorders, gastric ulcers, tissue repair, lung, stomach, esophagus, recurring ear infections, urinary infections, mouth, cervix, and colon cancer, angina, genital herpes, colds and flu, osteoarthritis, compromised immunity, HIV, Crohn's disease, diarrhea, heavy menstruation, peptic ulcer, and premenstrual syndrome

Scientific Updates: Vitamin A depletion may play a significant role in diseases like cancer, Crohn's disease and gastric ulcers. A recent study found that vitamin A supplementation reduces the incidence of night blindness better than beta-carotene alone.

Depletors: antibiotics, sulfa drugs, tobacco, contraceptive drugs, alcohol, cortisone, estrogen, mineral oil, coffee, some types of indoor lighting, air pollution

Safety: Most adults should not take over 25,000 IU of preformed vitamin A daily. More than this in either supplement form or in cod liver oil may result in toxicity causing possible headaches, blurred vision, hair loss, joint pain, dry skin, drowsiness, diarrhea, and enlargement of the liver and spleen. Pregnant women should not take over 5,000 IU daily. Taking beta-carotene alone cannot result in a vitamin A overdose. Do not take more than 5,000 IU daily if you are pregnant or trying to conceive. Plant-derived vitamin A precursors are considered nontoxic.

Special Instructions: For maximum absorption, take with foods containing some fat. Avoid taking with olestra-containing foods, high fiber meals or fiber supplements, which could impair absorption.

Product Availability: Vitamin C is available in capsules or softgels. It may also be combined with 400 to 1,000 IU of vitamin D. Beta-carotene or other mixed carotenoids may also be added to a vitamin A supplement.

References

Christian et al. 1998. Vitamin A or beta-carotene supplementation reduces but does not eliminate maternal night blindness in Nepal. *Journal of Nutrition* 128(9):1458–63.

Hepatogastroenterology. 1985. Jan-Feb. 32:34–38

Lancet. Oct. 16, 1982. p. 876.

The New England Journal of Medicine. 1984. 310: 1023–31

Vitamin D

Overview: Called the sunshine vitamin, ultraviolet rays convert a chemical found in the skin's surface to previtamin D3, which is eventually converted in the liver and kidneys into vitamin D. Vitamin D works to make calcium and phosphorus available to bones and teeth. For children whose bones are in the formative stage, adequate levels of vitamin D are crucial. Rickets, a disease characterized by a softening of the bones, is no longer a problem; however, low levels of vitamin D can contribute to osteomalacia or osteoporosis in older individuals.

Daily Value: 400 international units (10 micrograms)

Optimal Consumption: A daily dose of 600 IU for people over seventy is recommended, and up to 800 IU a day will benefit older people during dark winter months.

Applications: cancer prevention, melanoma, osteomalacia, osteoporosis, multiple sclerosis, Crohn's disease, fibromyalgia, muscle pain, epilepsy, high blood pressure, kidney disease, liver disease, SAD, skin aliments (psoriasis), type I diabetes prevention

Scientific Updates: A new study has found that vitamin D supplementation improves muscle strength and the ability to walk over distances in vitamin D-deficient older women. A deficiency of vitamin D plays a significant role in the development of type 1 (insulin-dependent) diabetes. Without enough vitamin D, islet cells of the pancreas don't produce insulin. Recent research suggests that elderly people may be deficient in this vitamin due to a lack of sunlight exposure and nutrient depletion. Studies have found that women are consistently low in vitamin D, which may predispose them to osteoporosis.

Depletors: mineral oil, smog, barbiturates, cholesterol lowering drugs, antacids, prednisone, anticonvulsive drugs, sedatives, intestinal disorders, liver/gallbladder disease, overuse of sunscreen, sunlight deprivation

Safety: Excessive doses (over 2,000 IU daily) taken for several months may cause high blood levels of calcium, kidney stones, and calcium deposits in heart and kidney tissues, which can be fatal. Calcium should always be taken with vitamin D. Most people should not exceed 1,000 IU a day.

Special Instructions: Take vitamin D with foods that contain some fat. It takes approximately 20 minutes of sunshine exposure daily on the hands and face to supply vitamin D. Keep in mind that UV sunblocks prohibit this action.

Product Availability: Vitamin D is available in 400 to 1,000 IU supplements and is sometimes combined with calcium and magnesium. Topical vitamin D ointments are used for psoriasis and skin rashes.

References

Clinical Science 1984. 66:103–07.

The Lancet Feb. 1985. 9:307–09.

Journal of the American College of Nutrition 1983. 2:73–99.

Journal of Clinical Nutrition 1982. 36:1225–33.

Journal of Bone and Joint Surgery 1982. p. 542–60.

Verhaai et al. 2000. Muscle strength, functional mobility and vitamin D in older women. *Aging* 12(6): 455–60.

Vitamin E

Overview: As one of nature's most potent antioxidants, vitamin E is found in the protective membranes of our cells and in the sheaths that protect our nerves. Because it so effectively scavenges for dangerous free radicals, it helps to prevent degenerative diseases including cancer. It also improves circulation and helps to repair damaged tissue. Vitamin E is considered an anti-aging nutrient in that it slows the tissue degeneration associated with free radical damage.

Daily Value: 30 IU

*1 mg alpha-tocopherol equivalents = 1.5 IU

Optimal Consumption: It is thought that optimal doses of vitamin E start at 100 IU. Keep in mind that if you are on a low fat diet, your intake can drop to 10 IU, making supplementation even more important. For people ages 45 and older, or for those with chronic diseases, optimal dosages range from 400 to 800 IU (consult safety section).

Applications: aging, angina, Alzheimer's disease, atherosclerosis, diabetes, heart disease, cancer, cataracts, fibrocystic breast disease, cholesterol, blood clots, rheumatoid arthritis, scar tissue, multiple sclerosis, PMS, infertility, impotence, leg cramps, lupus, cardiovascular disease, hypertension, burns, headaches, wound healing

Scientific Updates: European researchers have found that people with rheumatoid arthritis who take 800 IU a day of vitamin E reported less pain. Its anti-inflammatory effect may also help those with lupus, fibrocystic breast disease and fibromyalgia. Using it on the skin may also help to inhibit scarring.

Depletors: estrogen, birth control pills, mineral oil, chlorine, food processing, inorganic iron, rancid fat, faulty fat digestion, Crohn's disease

Safety: You should not use vitamin E if you are taking anticoagulants (blood thinners), ginkgo, fish-oil supplements or aspirin unless advised by your physician. Vitamin E should also be avoided if you have a history of stroke. If you have heart disease, consult with your doctor before taking vitamin E. Do not take iron at the same time as vitamin E. Anyone with hypertension, overactive thyroid, diabetes or rheumatic heart disease should not take excessive doses and begin with smaller doses with their doctor's approval. The Institute of Medicine has set an intake level for vitamin E at 1,000 mg (1,500 IU) for alpha-tocopherol varieties. Higher dosages can have an anticoagulant action and increase the risk of bleeding problems.

Special Instructions: Take with foods that contain some fat. There is evidence that natural forms (d-alpha tocopherol or d-alpha tocopheryl acetate or succinate) are better assimilated than synthetic products (dl-alpha tocopheryl acetate). The natural form can be twice as active and is retained for longer periods of time.

Product Availability: Vitamin E comes in D-alpha-tocopherol, d-alpha tocopheryl acetate, d-alpha tocopheryl succinate, and dl-alpha tocopheryl acetate forms. Natural vitamin E is also commonly combined with other forms, such as gamma tocopherol, that offer added protection. Other tocopherols such as this one are not present in synthetic vitamin E.

References

British Journal of Dermatology 1984. 3:125–26.

Canadian Journal of Neurological Science 1984. 2:561–64.

Journal of Nutrition 1986. 116:675–81.

Lancet 1983. 29:225–28.

Venkatraman, J. and W. Chu. 1999. Effects of dietary omega-3 and omega-6 lipids and vitamin E on serum cytokines, lipid mediators and anti-DNA antibodies in a mouse model for rheumatoid arthritis. *Journal of the American College of Nutrition* 18(6): 602–13.

Vitamin K *(Phylloquinone)*

Overview: Vitamin K is necessary for the production of several blood proteins required for clotting, including prothrombin. These proteins form clots to stop bleeding. A vitamin K deficiency would cause slow clotting resulting in frequent bruising or bleeding that is hard to stop. Vitamin K is also required to make certain proteins found in bone. Deficiencies in this vitamin can result in poor mineral absorption into bones making them weak and prone to fractures. Vitamin K also promotes a healthy liver and may prevent certain types of cancers.

Daily Value: 80 micrograms

Optimal Consumption: 100 micrograms

Applications: osteoporosis, hemorrhaging, heavy periods, post-surgery, colitis, gallstones

Scientific Updates: A study which found that a significant number of women who suffered from osteoporosis were also deficient in vitamin K suggests a link between the two. A new study supports the beneficial role of vitamin K supplementation to treat osteoporosis.

Depletors: antibiotics, premature birth, anticoagulant drugs, faulty fat absorption

Safety: If you are taking the anticoagulant warfarin (Coumadin) or other blood thinners, do not take vitamin K without medical supervision. You should not take large doses of synthetic vitamin K during pregnancy. Excessive doses can cause reddening of the skin and sweating. The development of hemolytic anemia may indicate a vitamin K overdose.

Special Instructions: Most people do not need vitamin K supplementation; however, if you suffer from heavy periods or gastrointestinal bleeding, you may benefit from vitamin K supplementation: For maximum absorption, take a vitamin K with a meal that contains some fat. Large intakes of vitamin E (over 2,000 IU) can reduce the absorption of vitamin K in the intestines.

Product Availability: Vitamin K is often added to other nutrients or can be purchased as a single supplement. It is also available in ointment form for the treatment of spider veins or bruises.

References

Journal of Clinical Endocrinology and Metabolism 1985. 60:1268–69.

Shearer, M. 2000. Role of vitamin K and GLA proteins in the pathophysiology of osteoporosis and vascular calcification. *Current Opinions in Clinical Nutritional Metabolism Care* 3(6):433–8.

Water-Soluble Vitamins

Vitamin B1 *(Thiamin)*

Overview: Thiamin helps to stimulate circulation and contributes to the production of blood and hydrochloric acid. It also takes part in the metabolism of carbohydrates. This vitamin is necessary for normal growth and the development of the muscles that line the gastrointestinal tract and comprise the heart. Thiamin supplementation fights mental deterioration associated with alcoholism and helps the brain use glucose. It is vital for proper energy usage and to prevent fatigue.

Applications: Alzheimer's disease, alcoholism, anemia, canker sores, depression, diarrhea, mental illness, stress, beriberi, shingles, infections, Wernicke-Korsakoff syndrome

Daily Value: 1.5 milligrams

Optimal Consumption: A thiamin deficiency is most likely to occur in people who diet excessively or abuse alcohol. Older individuals in nursing homes or hospitals can also become thiamin deficient.

Scientific Updates: An Israeli study found that 70 percent of people with recurring canker sores had low blood levels of thiamin. Thiamin deficiencies have also been linked to mental illness. Geriatric patients who have surgery may experience a thiamin loss, which may explain their postoperative confusion and mental deterioration. Antibiotics, oral contraceptives and sulfa drugs may also decrease thiamin levels. Eating a diet high in carbohydrates also increases the need for thiamin.

Depletors: stress, caffeine, alcohol, surgery, excess carbohydrate consumption (sugar), tobacco, raw fish and shellfish, antibiotics, oral contraceptives, sulfa drugs, muscle relaxants, excess dieting

Safety: Thiamin would have to be taken in inordinately large doses to produce any toxicity. There have been no reports of toxicity in human with oral supplements of vitamin B1.

Special Instructions: It's best to take the B-vitamins together to achieve the optimal synergistic effect. For optimal absorption, do not take this vitamin with coffee, tea or alcohol.

Product Availability: Thiamin is available as a single supplement and is also included in B-complex products.

References

Age and Aging 1982. 101–07.

British Journal of Psychiatry 1982. 141:271.

Haisraeli-Shalish et al. 1996. Recurrent aphthous stomatitis and thiamin deficiency. *Oral Surgery Oral Medicine Oral Pathol and Oral Radiology Endodontics* 82(6):634–6.

Journal of the American College of Nutrition 1988. 7:61–67.

Vitamin B2 *(Riboflavin)*

Overview: Vitamin B2 helps tproduce energy from consumed fats, carbohydrates, and protein. It also assists in the production of a powerful antioxidant called glutathione and must be present for the production of red blood cells. It prevents cataracts and facilitates the use of oxygen by certain body tissues. It also converts tryptophan (an amino acid) to niacin and maintains the mucous membranes of the intestinal tract.

Daily Value: 1.7 milligrams

Optimal Consumption: Health care practitioners may recommend higher doses for specific disease conditions.

Applications: anemia, arteriosclerosis, baldness, bladder infections, carpal tunnel, cataracts, hypoglycemia, immune system disorders, mental disorders, muscle diseases, morning sickness, obesity, sickle-cell anemia, stress, depression, trembling, migraine headaches

Scientific Updates: New studies suggest that riboflavin may help control migraines. Riboflavin deficiencies have been linked to cataract formation, psychiatric and emotional disorders, sickle cell anemia, and esophageal cancer. Some studies suggest that riboflavin therapy may help to alleviate carpal tunnel syndrome. Testing of forty-two adolescent boys found that 38 percent of them were riboflavin deficient.

Depletors: excessive dieting and exercise, diuretics, antibiotics, barbiturates, dialysis, alcohol, intestinal disorders, tobacco, oral contraceptives, coffee, cooking, radiation, ultraviolet light, white sugar, and estrogen

Safety: At high dosages, vitamin B2 may cause photosensitivity (skin rashes or burns when exposed to ultra-violet light).

Special Instructions: Riboflavin is very sensitive to light and can be destroyed. Purchase supplements in dark or opaque containers to preserve potency.

Product Availability: Vitamin B2 is commonly found in B-complex formulas and is also available as a single supplement.

References

American Journal of Clinical Nutrition. 1984. 39:787–91.

American Journal of Clinical Nutrition 1983. 38:884–87.

American Journal of Opthamology 1931. 14:1005–09.

Journal of the National Cancer Institute 1984. 72:941–48.

Proceedings of the National Academy of Science 1984. 81:7076–78.

Sandor et al. 2000. Prophylactic treatment of migraine with beta-blockers and riboflavin: differential effects on the intensity dependence of auditory evoked cortical potentials. *Headache* 0(1):30–5.

Vitamin B3 *(Niacin, Niacinamide, Nicotinic Acid)*

Overview: Vitamin B3 is necessary to release energy from carbohydrates. It is also required to process alcohol. In its niacin form, this vitamin helps your body regulate cholesterol.

Daily Value: 20 milligrams

Optimal Consumption: 10 to 25 mg of the vitamin can be taken as part of a B-complex or multivitamin supplement.

Applications: acne, anxiety, alcohol withdrawal, bursitis, cancer prevention, cataracts, diabetes, epilepsy, high cholesterol levels, high blood pressure, mental illness, migraines, leg cramps, poor circulation, intermittent claudication, postpartum support, Reynaud's disease, painful menstruation, stress, poor memory, senility

Scientific Updates: New analysis of niacin forms has concluded that it can be effectively used to treat high cholesterol with little toxicity and few side effects. Several clinical tests have confirmed the ability of niacin to lower blood cholesterol and triglycerides by up to 50 percent or more. Niacin has also proven its effectiveness in preventing cancer after exposure to carcinogens. Niacin may also be very useful for epilepsy and can be used in conjunction with anticonvulsant drugs.

Depletors: pregnancy, antibiotics, caffeine, alcohol, estrogen, sleeping pills, sulfa drugs and excessive consumption of white sugar

Safety: Niacinamide is considered quite safe, although rare liver problems have occurred at doses in excess of 1,000 mg per day. Niacin, in amounts as low as 50 to 100 mg, may cause flushing, headache, and stomachache in some people. Megadoses (over 1,000 mg daily) can cause liver damage, diabetes, gastritis, eye damage and elevated uric acid. After taking vitamin B3 a "niacin flush" may occur. This is a redness of the skin, usually in the face and neck region. A tingling sensation may also be experienced, but both of these reactions are harmless. Pregnant women or anyone with diabetes, gout, peptic ulcers, glaucoma, or liver ailments should not use high doses of vitamin B3. The inositol hexaniacinate form of niacin has not been linked with side effects; however, studies have been limited. Don't take this supplement in large amounts without the consent of your health care practitioner.

Special Instructions: Vitamin B3 works with vitamin B1 and B2 to release energy from carbohydrates. Therefore, these vitamins are often taken together in a B-complex or multiple vitamin supplement (although most B3 research uses niacin or niacinamide by itself).

Product Availability: Vitamin B3 comes in two forms: niacin (also called nicotinic acid) and niacinamide (also called nicotinamide). A variation of niacin called inositol hexaniacinate is also available. This form has fewer side effects and is sometimes prescribed for people who need stronger therapeutic doses of vitamin B3.

References

Drug Therapy 1984. p. 62–70.

Journal of the National Cancer Institute 1984. 73:767–70.

Knopp, R. 2000. Evaluating niacin in its various forms" *American Journal of Cardiology* 21:86(12 Suppl 1):51–56.

Vitamin B5 *(Pantothenic Acid)*

Overview: This B-vitamin has been called the anti-stress nutrient. It participates in the conversion of food to energy, the production of various hormones, and helps the body use fat and cholesterol. It also helps create lipoproteins, which comprise the very important membranes that surround our cells. Pantothenic acid also plays a vital role in the production of hemoglobin in red blood cells that makes the transport of oxygen throughout our bodies possible. It also detoxifies body tissues from dangerous chemicals.

Daily Value: 10 milligrams

Optimal Consumption:		
Infants	0 to 5 months, 1.7 mg
	6 to 11 months, 1.8 mg
Children	1 to 3 years, 2 mg
	4 to 8 years, 3 mg
	9 to 13 years, 4 mg
Adults	14 years and older, 4 mg

For lowering cholesterol and triglycerides, the typical recommended dosage of pantothenic acid is 300 mg three times daily. Dosages as high as 660 mg three times daily are sometimes recommended for people with arthritis. Both of these dosages require the consent of your health care practitioner.

Applications: alcoholism, anxiety, depression, allergies, anemia, arthritis, asthma, diabetes, Addison's disease, diarrhea, joint inflammation, high cholesterol, rheumatoid arthritis, menopausal symptoms, mental illness, muscle cramps, respiratory infections, stress, hair loss, premature aging

Scientific Updates: Pantetheine, a form of pantothenic acid in doses of 900 milligrams a day, has been shown to significantly reduce cholesterol and blood fats. It seems to inhibit the body's production of cholesterol while booting the utilization of fat for energy. Pantothenic acid in the form of calcium pantothenate (50 to 2,000 milligrams a day) has also been used to reduce the stiffness and pain of rheumatoid arthritis. Data reveals that some people suffering from rheumatoid arthritis have decreased levels of pantothenic acid. Using this vitamin therapeutically has resulted in the alleviation of typical arthritis symptoms in some people.

Depletors: insecticides, alcohol, coffee, cooking, sulfa drugs, estrogen, sleeping pills, cholesterol lowering drugs

Safety: No significant side effects have been reported for pantothenic acid or pantetheine, alone or in combination with other medications. However, maximum safe dosages for young children, pregnant or nursing women, or people with serious liver or kidney disease have not been established.

Special Instructions: Take with other B-vitamins for maximum effect.

Product Availability: Vitamin B5 is available as calcium pantothenate and pantetheine.

References

Biological Psychiatry 1984. 9:4:613–16.

Shimizu, S. 1999. Pantothenic acid. *Nippon Rinsho* 7(10):2218–22.

Vitamin B6 *(Pyridoxine)*

Overview: Vitamin B6 plays a primary role in the production of proteins, hormones, and neurotransmitters (chemicals that transmit signals between nerve cells). Deficiencies of this vitamin are common; in fact, in a survey of 11,658 adults, 71 percent of men and 90 percent of women were found to have diets deficient in B6. Vitamin B6 is the most commonly deficient water-soluble vitamin in the elderly and in children. New studies suggest that it can help prevent heart disease and ease the nausea typically seen in cases of morning sickness.

Daily Value: 2 milligrams

Optimal Consumption: Vitamin B6 requirements increase with age. Therapeutic doses can range into much higher levels; however, taking more than 50 mg daily is not advised unless under the supervision of your health care practitioner.

Applications: anxiety, carpal tunnel syndrome, depression, diabetic neuropathy, heart disease prevention, headaches, kidney disease, anemia, mental illness, hypoglycemia, epilepsy, arthritis, asthma, insomnia, Parkinson's disease, pregnancy, morning sickness, PMS, lactation, cataracts, eczema, high cholesterol, immune deficiency

Scientific Updates: Recent studies suggest that vitamin B6 supplementation can help alleviate the symptoms of PMS. A vitamin B6 deficiency has been profoundly linked to a number of mental disorders, including clinical depression and schizophrenia. Pyridoxine therapy has been successfully used to treat childhood autism, and epilepsy, has enhanced cardiovascular health and has inhibited melanoma in test animals. B6 depletion has also been connected to immune deficiency, kidney diseases, asthma, sickle cell anemia and diabetes.

Depletors: antidepressant drugs, alcohol, oral contraceptives, estrogen, most drugs, stress

Safety: Vitamin B6 appears to be safe for adults at dosages up to 50 mg daily. At higher dosages (over 200 mg) there is a significant risk of nerve damage. In some cases, high doses of vitamin B6 can cause or worsen acne and doses over 5 mg may interfere with the effects of the drug, levodopa. Safe dosages for children, pregnant or nursing women, or those with severe liver or kidney disease have not been established. If you are taking Isoniazid (INH), penicillamine, hydralazine, theophylline, or MAO inhibitors, you may need vitamin

B6 supplementation at normal dosages. Do not take more than 5 mg of vitamin B6 daily except on medical advice.

Special Instructions: The B vitamins work together, so taking B6 with other B vitamins is highly recommended. If you are taking various vitamin supplements that all contain B6, make sure you are not exceeding recommended levels.

Product Availability: Vitamin B6 is available as pyridoxine, pyridoxine hydrochloride, and pyridoxal-5-phosphate.

References

Annals of Neurology 1985. 17:117–20.

Atherosclerosis 1985. 55:357–61.

Biological Psychiatry 1984. 9:4:613–16.

Kant, A.K., and G. Block. 1990. Dietary vitamin B-6 intake and food sources in the US population: NHANES II, 1976–1980. *American Journal of Clinical Nutrition* 52:707–716.

Wyatt et al. 1999. Efficacy of vitamin B-6 in the treatment of premenstrual syndrome: systematic review. *British Medical Journal* 22:318(7195):1375–81.

Vitamin B12 *(Cyanocobalamin)*

Overview: This vitamin is essential for every cell process in your body. It must be available for DNA synthesis, the process by which your body makes the genetic materials that comprise the cell nucleus. Vitamin B12 helps make the nucleic acids that form DNA. It also helps make RNA, the copy of DNA that makes cell replication possible.

Daily Value: 6 micrograms

Optimal Consumption: Recommended doses of B12 should be adequate to correct mild deficiencies; however, therapeutic doses range from 100 to 2,000 mcg and should only be taken upon the advice of your health care practitioner.

Applications: mental disorders, depression, fatigue, pernicious anemia, male infertility, asthma, HIV support, Lou Gehrig's disease, diabetic neuropathy, multiple sclerosis, restless leg syndrome, tinnitus, Alzheimer's disease, osteoporosis, periodontal disease, shingles, hepatitis, neuritis, bursitis

Scientific Updates: Several studies support the notion that a vitamin B12 deficiency may account for psychiatric disturbances. A lack of this vitamin has also been linked to miscarriage and possible infertility. Using B12 in combination with other nutrients can also lower the risk of glaucoma.

Note: Vitamins B6, B12 and folic acid can lower blood levels of homocysteine to reduce risk of heart attack and prevent intermittent claudication, phlebitis, Alzheimer's disease, angina and high blood pressure.

Depletors: anticoagulant drugs, anti-gout medication, laxatives, alcohols, aspirin, antibiotics, diuretics, antacids, caffeine, Crohn's disease, strict vegetarianism, estrogen, sleeping pills, contraceptives, high cooking temperatures. Note: Elderly people and vegetarians are susceptible to vitamin B12 deficiencies due to low levels of stomach acid.

Safety: While it is generally regarded as safe, high doses of B12 can cause or worsen acne. If you are taking medications that reduce stomach acid such as H2 blockers; e.g., Zantac (ranitidine) and proton pump inhibitors; e.g., Prilosec (omeprazole), colchicine and AZT, you may need extra B12. Prolonged exposure to nitrous oxide may result in a type of anemia caused by a lack of vitamin B12.

Special Instructions: People with B12 deficiencies may need B12 injections as well as other supplementation. Because the B vitamins tend to work together, many nutritional experts recommend taking B12 with other B vitamins in the form of a B-complex supplement.

Product Availability: Vitamin B12 is also available as methylcobalamin, cyanocobalamin, hydrocobalamin, or cobalamin. Using sub-lingual forms of this vitamin help to ensure its assimilation. Certain forms of brewer's yeast provide a vegetarian source of vitamin B12.

References

Bennett, M. 2001. Vitamin B12 deficiency, infertility and recurrent fetal loss. *Journal of Reproductive Medicine* 46(3):209–12.

British Journal of Psychiatry 1988. 153:266–67.

Head, K. 2001. Natural therapies for ocular disorders, part two: cataracts and glaucoma. *Alternative Medicine Review* 6(2):141–166.

Biotin

Overview: Biotin is a nutrient and member of the B-vitamin family that not only thickens and fortifies brittle nails, but also assists the body in using carbohydrates, fat, and protein to produce energy needed to fuel body systems. It also helps in tissue regeneration and is particularly vital to newborns. Biotin may also be beneficial for diabetics.

Daily Value: 300 micrograms or 0.3 milligrams

Optimal Consumption: Same as daily value

Applications: thin brittle nails, seborrheic dermatitis, diabetes, baldness, depression, eczema, leg cramps

Scientific Updates: In new studies, biotin supplementation boosted the action of insulin in controlling blood sugar and may help to prevent type II diabetes. New research has also found that, with biotin supplementation, people on dialysis may see significant improvement in neurological disorders suffered as a result of kidney treatment. One study found that an additional 2,500 micrograms a day of biotin helped to strengthen and thicken brittle fingernails. Biotin is necessary to make keratin, which comprises hair and nails.

Depletors: raw egg whites, sulfa drugs, saccharin, rancid fats, refined foods, estrogen, white sugar, alcohol, Crohn's disease. Note: The presence of seborrheic dermatitis in infants may indicate a biotin deficiency.

Safety: Biotin is considered nontoxic.

Special Instructions: Take in divided doses with meals. You need only a tiny amount of biotin: 300 micrograms, or about one-third of a milligram daily to achieve therapeutic effects.

Product Availability: Two excellent sources of biotin are royal jelly, a substance secreted by bees, and brewer's yeast.

References

McCarty, M. 2000. Toward practical prevention of type 2 diabetes. *Medical Hypotheses* 54(5):786–93.

Nephron. 36, 1984, 183–86.

Sone, H. 2000. Characteristics of the biotin enhancement of glucose-induced insulin release in pancreatic islets of the rat. *Bioscience Biotechnology Biochemistry* 64(3):550–4.

Choline

Overview: This nutrient is part of the vitamin B complex family and acts as a precursor for acteylcholine, a brain chemical necessary for the proper transmission of messages between nerve cells. Choline also helps prevent fat accumulation in the liver and works in tandem with inositol to metabolize fats and cholesterol. Choline is vital for proper memory and learning functions. The body can manufacture choline when vitamin B12, folic acid and methionine (an amino acid) are present.

Daily Value: none assigned

Applications: Parkinson's disease, early Alzheimer's disease, liver disorders, gallstones, heart disease, memory loss, depression, stress, high cholesterol, arteriosclerosis, baldness, multiple sclerosis, glaucoma, eczema, alcoholism, muscular dystrophy, hypertension, diseases of the nervous system

Scientific Updates: In a very recent study, choline supplementation significantly improved both verbal and visual memory skills in test groups with impaired brain function, which suggests its potential in early cases of Alzheimer's disease. Studies have also shown that taking lecithin (a good source of choline) can decrease cholesterol levels and may be an effective way to treat atherosclerosis.

Depletors: water, sulfa drugs, estrogen, food processing, alcohols, excess sugar consumption

Safety: Choline has no known side effects. However, very large doses may produce nausea, dizziness or diarrhea. Large doses of lecithin that contain choline may also cause upset stomach, sweating, salivation and loss of appetite. Don't take choline in doses above 3.5 grams without the consent of your doctor.

Special Instructions: If you choose choline bitartrate, use it in small amounts initially as it can cause diarrhea. Choline is available in tablet form and may cause you to emit a fishy smell. Taking lecithin as a choline source does not result in this effect.

Product Availability: Supplemental choline is available in lecithin (phosphatidyl choline) capsules and granules. Choline chloride or choline bitartrate is also available; choline is also found in brewer's yeast.

References
Biochemical and Medical Metabolism and Biology 1986. Jan-Feb:31–39.

Buchman et al. 2001. Verbal and visual memory improve after choline supplementation in long-term total parenteral nutrition: a pilot study. *Journal of Parenteral and Enteral Nutrition* 25(1):30–5.

Folic Acid *(Folate, folacin)*

Overview: Folic acid is essential for the production of DNA and RNA which permits cell to replicate, making it a crucial nutrient during pregnancy. A lack of folic acid has been linked to birth defects. Deficiencies may also cause anemia, nutrient absorption problems and heart disease.

Daily Value: 400 micrograms

Optimal Consumption: Most people only obtain an average of 200 micrograms of folate daily. The majority of multivitamins contain 400 micrograms and prenatal vitamins can contain 800 micrograms.

Applications: alcoholism, anemia, arteriosclerosis, birth defect prevention, baldness, cervical cancer, diarrhea, depression, gout, gingivitis, heart disease, mental illness, mental retardation, immune system, birth defect prevention, fatigue, ulcers, stress, blood disorders

Scientific Updates: New analysis of folate supplementation points to its potential value for Alzheimer's disease, and for the prevention of heart disease. It is also being investigated for its beneficial effects on several cancers and on mood disorders. Numerous studies support the use of folic acid supplementation during and after pregnancy to prevent birth defects and postpartum depression.

Depletors: oral contraceptives, high heat, dieting, blood loss, measles and chicken pox, malabsorption, alcohol, stress, coffee, sulfa drugs, tobacco, estrogen, barbiturates, cholestryramine, dilantin.

Note: A tongue that is red and sore may indicate a folic acid deficiency.

Safety: Anyone with hormonally-related cancers or with convulsive disorders should not use excessive amounts of folic acid for extended periods of time. Because folic acid supplementation lowers plasma zinc levels, women who are taking oral contraceptives (which also lower zinc) may become zinc deficient. Do not take doses above 1,000 micrograms a day without medical supervision.

Special Instructions: The daily value of folic acid for pregnant women is 800 micrograms daily.

Product Availability: Folic acid is usually included in multiple formulas but is also available as a separate supplement. Make sure your multiple offers a minimum of the daily value.

References

The Lancet 1982. 24: 217.

Lucock, M. and I. Daskalakis. 2000. New perspectives on folate status: a differential role for the vitamin in cardiovascular disease, birth defects and other conditions. *British Journal of Biomedicine and Science* 57(3):254–60.

Inositol

Overview: Inositol is a fatty lipid that is required for cell membrane formation. It is sometimes referred to as vitamin B8. It is most abundantly found in the heart and brain, and it directly affects nerve transmission and participates in the transportation of fats throughout the body. Most dietary inositol is in the form of phytate.

Daily Value: none assigned

Optimal Consumption: Although many think most people do not need inositol supplementation, nutrition experts often suggest 500 mg twice per day for diabetic neuropathy and doses up to 12 grams per day have been used for neuropsychiatric problems. Your doctor should approve doses greater than 500 mg.

Applications: anxiety, baldness, depression, diabetes, diabetic neuropathy, eczema, psoriasis, cardiovascular disease, arteriosclerosis, cirrhosis of the liver, glaucoma, panic disorders, obesity, gallbladder disease, multiple sclerosis, mental disorders

Scientific Updates: New studies suggest that inositol may help infants who suffer from respiratory distress syndrome. A 2000 review found it helped prevent adverse effects normally seen after respiratory distress syndrome. Inositol also helps remove fats from the liver, is vital for the formation of lecithin and helps properly maintain cholesterol levels in the blood. It can also help to elevate mood and fight depression.

Depletors: caffeine, alcohols, insecticides, sulfa drugs, diabetes

Safety: Considered safe if not used in excess. People with chronic kidney failure show elevated levels of inositol. No long-term safety studies have been performed and its safety has not been established in young children, women who are pregnant or nursing, and those with severe liver and kidney disease.

Special Instructions: Diabetics have an increased excretion of inositol and may need supplementation.

Product Availability: Some inositol supplements have a dairy base and should not be used by anyone with lactose intolerance.

References

Howlett, A. and A. Ohlsson. 2000. Inositol for respiratory distress syndrome in preterm infants. *Cochrane Database System Review* 4(4):CD000366.

Levine, J. 1997. Controlled trials of inositol in psychiatry. *European Neuropsychopharmacology* 7:147–155.

PABA *(Para-Aminobenzoic Acid)*

Overview: Some nutritionists consider PABA a member of the vitamin B-complex family although its properties differ from other B-vitamins. PABA is thought to enhance the effects of cortisone, and it may help to reverse the buildup of abnormal fibrous tissue. It is also vital to the production of folic acid in the body.

Daily Value: none assigned

Optimal Consumption: Therapeutic doses of PABA range from 300 mg per day up to 12 grams per day for autoimmune or connective tissue disorders. Anyone taking more than 400 mg of PABA per day should consult their health care practitioner.

Applications: connective tissue disorders, eczema, nervous disorders, baldness, hyperthyroidism, scleroderma, stress, infertility, Peyronie's disease. *Note:* PABA supplements have been known to restore gray hair to its original color in animals; however, in humans this has not been substantiated.

Scientific Updates: PABA is included in sunscreens for its ability to block ultraviolet rays. Taking PABA orally cannot prevent sunburn.

Depletors: coffee, alcohols, estrogen, sulfa drugs, food processing

Safety: No serious side effects have been reported with 300 to 400 mg per day. Larger doses (over 8 grams) may cause low blood sugar, low white cell count, rash, fever, and (on rare occasions) liver damage and vitiligo. The ingestion of 20 grams in small children can be fatal. PABA interferes with sulfa drugs (a class of antibiotics) and therefore should not be taken when these medications are being used.

Special Instructions: Most nutritionists do not consider PABA an essential nutrient. Small amounts of PABA are present in some B-complex vitamins and multi-vitamin formulas. If you are treating a specific disorder, you should purchase it as a separate supplement and take it according to the specifications of your health care practitioner.

Product Availability: Look for hypo-allergenic products that contain no yeast, dairy, egg, gluten, corn, soy or wheat if you have food sensitivities. Most products come in 100 mg tablets.

Vitamin C *(Ascorbic Acid)*

Overview: Vitamin C is a water-soluble vitamin that has powerful antioxidant actions. It contributes to the formation of collagen, the substance that gives strength to skin, muscles and blood vessels. It also plays a role in wound healing, fights infection, acts as a natural antihistamine and helps to detoxify the body of dangerous poisons. New research confirms its ability to help clear arteries of dangerous forms of cholesterol. Due to other properties, it is considered a very heart healthy vitamin and may prevent the formation of cataracts.

Daily Value: 60 milligrams

Optimal Consumption: A minimum of 500 to 1,000 mg of vitamin C per day is considered optimal by many health practitioners. Greater doses (up to 10,000 mg per day) are not uncommon. There is some speculation that doses above 200 mg are excreted in the urine and serve no purpose. Fatigue, easy bruising, and bleeding gums are early signs of vitamin C deficiency that can occur in elderly individuals Smokers also have lower levels of vitamin C and require a higher daily intake to maintain normal levels.

Applications: infections, bladder infections, bronchitis, bruising, capillary fragility, cataracts, colds and flu, diabetes, immune function, gallstones, gingivitis, glaucoma, sinusitis, earaches, sore throats, smokers, blood clots, atherosclerosis, high blood pressure, high cholesterol, physical and mental stress, weak immune system, liver toxicity, wound healing

Scientific Updates: Although the debate as to whether vitamin C supplementation can prevent colds continues, it can reduce the duration and severity of a cold. Megadoses of vitamin C (1 to 10 grams daily) taken at the onset of a cold can shorten its length. Numerous studies have also proven the ability of vitamin C to help open constricted bronchiole tubes, accelerate wound healing, prevent cataracts, scavenge free radicals and help prevent cardiovascular disease. Its role in cancer prevention is also thought to be significant. New data shows that low levels of vitamin C in people with head injuries are linked to more brain damage.

Depletors: aspirin, alcohol, antidepressant drugs, analgesics, oral contraceptives, anticoagulants, steroids, cooking, food processing, diuretics, air pollution, smoking, acetaminophen toxicity

Safety: Vitamin C is considered nontoxic. Some studies suggest that taking it in large doses depletes vitamin B12 stores and may be linked to cell mutation. Anyone who has a history of kidney stones should take vitamin C only with a physician's approval. Unusually excessive doses may cause intestinal upset, gas or diarrhea. Pregnant or nursing mothers should not use amounts larger than 5,000 milligrams daily. High levels of vitamin C can deplete the body of copper. Vitamin C may also increase the absorption of iron and helps to recycle vitamin E.

People with the following conditions should consult their doctor before supplementing with vitamin C:

- cancer
- glucose-6-phosphate dehydrogenase deficiency
- iron overload (hemosiderosis or hemochromatosis)

- history of kidney stones
- kidney failure

Vitamin C may inhibit the effect of the following substances:

- anti-cholinergics
- oral anticoagulants
- copper
- Megadoses of vitamin C increase chance of formation of drug crystals in urine if combined with aminosalicylic acid (PAS for tuberculosis).

Depletors: aspirin, tobacco, barbiturates, mineral oil, oral contraceptives, salicylates, sulfa drugs, tetracyclines

Special Instructions: Some experts recommend limiting the consumption of chewable vitamin C tablets because they can cause enamel loss on the teeth.

Product Availability: Although there are now several forms of vitamin C available (time released, buffered, etc.) using plain ascorbic acid can be effective and much less expensive. In its powdered form, it can be easily added to liquids. If you use ascorbic acid, add a bioflavonoid supplement to enhance its absorption and action. Combination vitamin C products derived from rose hips and other natural sources are also available.

References

American Review of Respiratory Disease. 1983. 127:143–47.

Douglas et al. 2000. Vitamin C for preventing and treating the common cold. *Cochrane Database System Review* 3(2): CD000980.

Oral Surgery. March 1982.

Polidori et al. 2001. Plasma vitamin C levels are decreased and correlated with brain damage in patients with intracranial hemorrhage or head trauma. *Stroke* 32(4):898–902.

Vitamin P *(Bioflavonoids)*

Overview: Although they technically are not vitamins, over 64 varieties of bioflavonoids are found in the white portion of citrus fruit peel, as well as in pine bark and grape seed. Bioflavonoids act as antioxidants and natural anti-inflammatory agents. Some of the better-known ones include hesperidin, rutin, and quercitin and help to make Vitamin C more available to the body. They also have impressive anti-inflammatory properties, strengthen capillary walls, and discourage bruising. Their primary benefit may be their protection of vitamin C from oxidation.

Daily Value: none assigned

Optimal Consumption: There is no recommended daily dosage for bioflavonoids. If you are treating a specific condition, you may want to take more than the amount included with your vitamin C supplement. Typically, if you have a particular condition, suggested dosages are 1,000 mg of citrus bioflavonoids or 400 mg of quercitin, each taken three times daily.

Applications: bruising, varicose veins, spider veins, arthritis, hemorrhaging, cholesterol levels, herpes, diabetes, diabetic retinopathy, cataracts, inflammation, phlebitis, bleeding gums, blood clots, colds, cold sores, scurvy, hemorrhoids, edema, hypertension, hemophilia

Scientific Updates: New studies have found that quercitin can protect cells against the damaging effects of ultraviolet light. Studies have also shown that quercitin can reduce cold sores and may ease allergy symptoms by strengthening cell walls that leak during allergic reactions. Bioflavonoids may also deactivate an enzyme called aldose reductase, which leads to cataracts.

Depletors: aspirin, alcohol, cortisone, antibiotics, smoking, some pain killing drugs

Safety: Bioflavonoids are considered nontoxic.

Special Instructions: Even if you are taking bioflavonoids as a separate supplement, combine them with vitamin C for optimal effects.

Product Availability: Quercetin can be purchased as a single supplement in capsule form, although bioflavonoid combinations are more common. Rutin is often added to vitamin C supplements to boost its effectiveness. Many vitamin C supplements contain bioflavonoids, which work to enhance the action and absorption of the vitamin.

References

Erden, M. and A. Kahraman. 2000. The protective effect of flavonol quercitin against ultraviolet a induced oxidative stress in rats. *Toxicology* 23:154(1–3):21–9.

Multi-Talented Minerals

Like vitamins, minerals function as coenzymes. They enable the body to carry out virtually every biochemical reaction needed to sustain life. Minerals are naturally occurring elements that come from soil, rock, water, animal and plant sources. Minerals can be classified as "macro" or "bulk" minerals, and "micro" or "trace" minerals. Bulk minerals, which are needed in more substantial amounts, include calcium, magnesium, potassium, phosphorus and sodium. Trace minerals include zinc, copper, iron, manganese, chromium, selenium and iodine. These are only needed in tiny amounts.

Mineral Mania

Today more than ever, we need to be taking mineral supplementation seriously. Agricultural practices have resulted in mineral-depleted foods that look beautiful but can be significantly mineral deficient. Intensive farming methods have depleted nutrients from our soils, which suggests that a diet rich in fresh foods does not guarantee a diet high in minerals and vitamins. Remember that a vegetable cannot be rich in minerals if it grew in low mineral soils. Estimates point out that farm soils in most of the world's agricultural regions are deficient in almost 85 percent of all minerals. Chemical fertilizers such as nitrogen, phosphorus and potassium can make plants grow rapidly; however, they do not replace the full array of minerals contained in in rich soil.

Depleted Soil Lacks Minerals

Statistics from the 1992 Earth Summit indicate that the mineral content of the world's farm and range soil has decreased dramatically.

Percentage of Mineral Depletion from Soil during the Past 100 Years, by Continent:

North America	85%
South America	76%
Asia	76%
Africa	74%
Europe	72%
Australia	55%

Keep in mind that without the presence of minerals, vitamins could not function properly in the human body. Studies tell us that iron, calcium and selenium deficiencies are much too common in certain segments of our population. Because our seemingly beautiful produce may be mineral deficient due to mineral-poor soil, supplementation is a good idea.

In an issue of *August Celebration*, Linda Grover made a very enlightening and somewhat alarming statement. She said, "In 1948 you could buy spinach that had 158 milligrams of iron per hundred grams. By 1965, the maximum iron they could find had dropped to 27 milligrams. In 1973, it was averaging 2.2. That's down from a hundred and fifty. That means today you'd have to eat 75 bowls of spinach to get the same amount of iron that one bowl might have given you back in 1948."

We need to replenish these vital minerals in supplement form. We not only need nitrogen and potassium to survive, but chromium, calcium, magnesium, copper, iron, molybdenum, cobalt, iodine and many other trace minerals as well. Commenting on the current mineral situation of our produce supply, Dr. Michael Colgan, who wrote, *The New Nutrition* stated, "Unfortunately, the human body cannot create minerals, so it has to get them through dietary means. Hence, deficient food produces deficient bodies (which culminates in sickness and disease)."

The Meaning of "Chelated" Minerals

Minerals attached to a molecule of protein that enhances their transportation into the bloodstream are called chelated. Chelated minerals are thought to be more absorbable and are recommended for any mineral supplementation. As with vitamins, a balanced array of minerals should be taken in order to achieve optimal results. Taking minerals with meals also helps to make them more absorbable.

Note: Increased dietary fiber can deplete mineral supplies if high dosages are used. Make sure to take a good mineral supplement at a different time than the fiber in order to avoid this effect.

What Are Trace Minerals?

Strange sounding compounds like nickel, molybdenum, germanium, manganese and vanadium belong to a class of nutrients called trace minerals. Like copper, iron and chromium, these minerals are only needed in tiny amounts to perform biological functions. In many instances, these trace minerals activate the actions of enzymes, which initiate and control virtually every chemical reaction in the human body. At this writing, many trace minerals still need evaluation to determine amounts needed by the body. We do know that using these minerals in therapeutic dosages has had some promising results for the treatment of several diseases.

A Word on Iron

Unless you suffer from an iron-deficiency, you probably don't need an iron-containing supplement. Excess iron levels have been linked to increased risk of heart attack and atherosclerosis and pose a significant health hazard to children.

Individual Mineral Profiles

Boron *(Trace mineral)*

Overview: Boron is a trace mineral that may soon be listed as essential. It maintains calcium balance, keeping bones strong and preventing osteoporosis. It may also prevent high blood pressure and certain forms of arthritis. In the human body, the highest concentrations of boron are found around the parathyroid gland. Boric acid is made from boron and has been used as an astringent and antiseptic.

Daily Value: none assigned

Optimal Consumption: No one knows how much boron we need. Estimates place need at between 3 and 5 mg daily.

Applications: malnutrition (elderly), osteoporosis, postmenopause

Scientific Updates: Boron supplementation shows promise for menopausal women who need to retain calcium to prevent osteoporosis. Boron may also play a role in high blood pressure and arthritis due to its link to calcium metabolism. More research in these areas is needed.

Depletors: Boron depletion is relatively rare.

Safety: More than three milligrams per day is not recommended.

Special Instructions: It is thought that 3 to 5 mg of boron is needed to maintain healthy bones. It's not uncommon to find Boron added to bone formulas containing calcium. Elderly people at risk for osteoporosis should take 1 to 3 mg of boron daily. Studies also suggest that 3 to 5 mg of boron daily can improve calcium retention in postmenopausal women.

Product Availability: Boron can be purchased as a separate supplement but is most often added to calcium/magnesium formulas. More multivitamin and mineral formulas are also adding 1 to 2 mg of boron to their formulas.

References

Hunt et al. 1997. Metabolic responses of postmenopausal women to supplemental dietary boron and aluminum during usual and low magnesium intake: boron, calcium, and magnesium absorption and retention and blood mineral concentrations. *American Journal of Clinical Nutrition* 65(3):803–13.

Calcium

Overview: Calcium is the most plentiful mineral in the human body and one of the most important. Vital for strong bones and teeth and to maintain regular heartbeat, calcium also lowers the risk of colon cancer and protects against osteoporosis. Vitamin D, magnesium and certain hormones must be present for calcium absorption and function. It is estimated that approximately 30 percent of our population eats calcium-deficient diets, which is one reason osteoporosis is so prevalent. Postmenopausal women and the elderly are prone to calcium deficiencies.

Daily Value: 800 to 1,000 milligrams

Optimal Consumption: How much calcium you need depends on your particular situation. It is thought that due to our high protein diets, 800 mg of calcium may not be enough to prevent osteoporosis. Calcium absorption usually decreases with age. If you increase your calcium intake, you should also increase magnesium intake, to one-half the calcium supply. Magnesium helps calcium stay more soluble, and thereby may reduce the risk of kidney stone formation and other calcifications. For phosphorus, an intake of about 800 to 1,000 mg is recommended when the calcium intake is 1,000 to 1,200 mg.

Applications: high blood pressure, osteoporosis prevention and treatment, PMS, menopause, pregnancy, lactation, nervous conditions, hyperactivity, restless leg syndrome, muscle cramping, insomnia, colon cancer protection, heart arrhythmia, periodontal disease, fractures, people taking Synthroid

Scientific Updates: New studies have found that calcium supplementation over an extended period of time can significantly improve symptoms associated with PMS. The World Health Organization recently developed a new definition of osteoporosis. They defined low bone mass as bone mineral density more than 1 standard deviation (SD) below the young normal mean. Women with bone density levels more than 2.5 SD below the young normal mean are presumed to have osteoporosis. It is estimated that 16.8 million postmenopausal white women (50 years of age) in this country have low bone mass, and 9.4 million actually have osteoporosis.

Depletors: pregnancy and nursing, low stomach hydrochloric acid, lack of exercise, stress, foods high in oxalic acid, sugar, high fiber foods, high protein diets, various metabolic disorders

Safety: Calcium is considered safe, however, anyone with kidney disease, kidney stones or who takes calcium channel blocking drugs should not take calcium without the consent of their physician. A high calcium intake for short periods of time is considered safe, as excesses are usually eliminated. Keep in mind that high calcium doses can cause constipation. If you take high doses, make sure to also take magnesium and vitamin D. Taking high amounts of calcium for long periods can lead to abnormal calcification of long bones in children or to hypercalcemia (high blood calcium levels) and soft tissue calcification in adults. If parathyroid weakness exists, calcium can accumulate.

Special Instructions: Taking vitamin D and magnesium in combination with calcium enhances assimilation and function. It's wise to take two smaller doses at separate times. Calcium citrate, lactate or gluconate can be taken between meals. All other forms of supplemental calcium are best absorbed when taken with food. Avoid taking calcium with any kind of bran. A diet excessively high in protein can interfere with calcium absorption. In addition, foods high in oxalic acid, such as spinach, rhubarb and chocolate, can interfere with calcium absorption. Moreover, an excessive use of antacids can prevent calcium absorption. Phytic acid, or phytates, found in whole grain foods or high fiber foods may also decrease the absorption of calcium and other minerals. Exposure to the sun increases the production of vitamin D thereby improving the absorption of calcium. Taking a calcium supplement directly after sunbathing can improve its utilization.

Product Availability: Calcium supplements come as calcium carbonate, citrate, citrate-malate, lactate, gluconate aspartate, dicalcium phosphate, bone meal, oyster shell and dolomite. Calcium chelates are available as calcium aspartate or calcium citrate and have a high rate of absorption. One of the drawbacks of bone meal or oyster shell is possible lead contamination. Many experts turn to aspartate or citrate salts of calcium. Chelated calcium supplements with amino acids are also easily absorbed. Calcium gluconate is another good choice.

References

Thys-Jacobs et al. 1998. Calcium carbonate and the premenstrual syndrome: effects on premenstrual and menstrual symptoms. *American Journal of Obstetrics and Gynecology* 179(2):444–452.

Chromium *(trace mineral)*

Overview: Discovered in 1957, chromium is considered a real trace mineral because so little is needed. For example, human blood contains approximately twenty parts per billion of chromium. Despite the tiny amounts required, chromium is vital to health maintenance. We now know that higher tissue levels of chromium are linked to a lower incidence of diabetes and atherosclerosis. In countries where the soil is rich in chromium, people have less heart and blood sugar diseases Chromium is an essential part of glucose tolerance factor (GTF); a molecule that regulates carbohydrate metabolism by enhancing insulin function. It also plays a role in cholesterol production

Daily Value: 120 to 200 micrograms

Optimal Consumption: Very few people get the daily value of 120 micrograms (mcg) of chromium. Studies show that the average diet contains about 25 mcg of chromium. To ensure optimal tissue levels, we need to consume a minimum of 100 to 200 mcg per day. Consequently, a better supplemental dose of chromium should fall between 200 and 300 mcg. The majority of multiple vitamin and mineral supplements contain 100 to 150 mcg of chromium. For various disorders, some health care experts recommend taking up to 1,000 mcg (1 mg) daily for short periods of time. If you have diabetes, the upper limits are 400 to 600 mcg daily, and you will need to carefully monitor your blood sugar levels while taking the supplement. Never discontinue the use of insulin or any other medication without the approval of your physician.

Applications: blood sugar disorders (type I and II diabetes, glucose intolerance, insulin resistance, hypoglycemia), binge eating, heart disease, high cholesterol, obesity

Scientific Updates: A new study confirms that chromium supplements can help to improve insulin resistance; a condition linked to obesity and heart disease. Asian trials support the use of chromium picolinate for type II diabetes.

Depletors: high sugar diets, diabetes, insulin resistance, infections, injuries

Safety: Don't take over 200 mcg a day without the consent of your health care practitioner. If you suffer from diabetes or hypoglycemia, consult your physician prior to taking a chromium supplement. Keep in mind that if you suffer from low blood sugar, symptoms of hypoglycemia may appear if chromium is taken in excess.

Special Instructions: Scientists believe chromium is better absorbed when taken with niacin, glycine, cysteine and glutamic acid.

Product Availability: Chromium comes in the following types: picolinate, nicotinate, aspartate, chloride and what may be labeled GTF chromium. Chromium chloride is the least absorbable form. GTF chromium is a combination of chromium, nicotinic acid and amino acids, which may vary in its composition.

References
Morris et al. 1998. Chromium supplementation improves insulin resistance in patients with Type II diabetes mellitus. *Nutrition Review* 56(10):302-6.

Copper *(Trace Mineral)*

Overview: Copper contributes to healing, the synthesis of hemoglobin and the production of hair and skin color. Copper is also essential for collagen formation. Copper-containing enzymes have several biological roles. They contribute to the formation of connective tissue, help to produce energy, make cholesterol and help the body use iron. Without copper, our heart, liver, kidneys, thyroid and immune systems would not function properly. There is also some evidence that copper helps to prevent osteoporosis and keeps cholesterol levels in check.

Daily Value: 2 milligrams

Optimal Consumption: Most people consume less than 1.5 milligrams of copper daily from food. Because this is less than the recommended daily value of 2 mg, you can either choose a supplement that includes copper or increase your consumption of copper-containing foods.

Applications: bacterial, viral and fungal infections, high cholesterol, poor hair growth, osteoporosis

Scientific Updates: Several international studies show that a lack of copper raises cholesterol levels in laboratory test animals. When copper levels are low, an enzyme called HMG-coA reductase in the liver becomes overly activated and as a result, cholesterol goes up. For this reason, the use of copper to prevent and treat atherosclerosis is currently under review.

Depletors: excess vitamin C and zinc, excess fructose, a diet high in white sugar

Safety: An excess of copper can create a vitamin C and zinc deficiency. The opposite is also true: taking high amounts of zinc or vitamin C can lower copper levels. Too much supplemental copper can cause health problems. Signs of excess copper include vomiting and diarrhea. Taking less than 10 milligrams occasionally is considered safe, but do not take more than 2 milligrams on a regular basis. Consult your doctor before taking higher amounts.

Special Instructions: It's best to take copper as part of a multiple vitamin and mineral supplement. Look for products that contain up to 2 milligrams of copper. Keep in mind that vitamin C interferes with copper absorption and assimilation. Don't take over 100 mg of vitamin C with a copper containing supplement for maximum effect.

Product Availability: Copper is rarely taken as a single supplement and is usually included in multiple formulas.

References
Lamb et al. 1999. Dietary copper supplementation reduces atherosclerosis in the cholesterol-fed rabbit. *Atherosclerosis* 146(1):33-43.

Germanium *(Trace mineral)*

Overview: Recently discovered by Japanese scientists, germanium is an effective antioxidant. Organic germanium can increase tissue oxygenation and is naturally found in the soil and in some plants. Although science does not consider germanium an essential mineral, new studies suggest that its powerful antioxidant action may be useful in many health conditions. Organic germanium sesquioxide (Ge-132) has been shown to boost the flow of oxygen flow to tissues and to enhance the function of immune-boosting cells. It may also treat viral infections, including AIDS, and chronic fatigue disorders. The Japanese use germanium as an overall tonic.

Daily Value: none assigned

Optimal Consumption: Because no one really know how much germanium is needed for optimal health, most experts advise moderate doses ranging from 50 to 150 mg.

Applications: rheumatism, cataracts, arthritis, immune dysfunction, high cholesterol, infections, chronic fatigue syndrome, viral infections, food allergies, pain, liver diseases, allergies and cancer

Scientific Updates: Studies suggest that Ge-132 can help to prevent the progress of cataracts and reduce pain in people with terminal cancer. This form of germanium actually inhibits the protein changes that take place when blood sugar is high, causing cataracts. This study suggests that germanium supplementation may be of special benefit to anyone with diabetes who may be at higher risk for blindness or cataract formation.

Depletors: none identified

Safety: Very few side effects have been associated with common dosages of germanium and its toxicity is considered low to none. Some serious side effects have been reported with germanium dioxide. Ge-132 organic germanium is considered safe if taken as directed.

Special Instructions: Do not use germanium dioxide, because, unlike organic forms, it has been associated with serious side effects.

Product Availability: You can find organic germanium compounds in loose powder form or capsulized form and range from 25 to 150 mg in potency. Organic germanium supplements are typically quite expensive. Japanese researchers have developed synthetic germanium compounds, whose therapeutic effects are reported to be more dramatic than natural sources. Organic germanium sesquioxide, also known as Ge-132 is one of these compounds.

References

Unakar, N. et al. 1997. Effect of pretreatment of germanium-132 on Na(+)-K(+)-ATPase and galactose cataracts. *Current Eye Research* 16(8):832–7.

Iodine

Overview: Iodine is famous for its role in the production of thyroid hormone. Almost all of the iodine contained in the body is found in the thyroid gland. Thyroid hormones control metabolic rate and regulate the way the body uses energy and stores fat. Decades ago, iodine deficiencies resulted in a condition called a goiter which caused the thyroid gland to become severely enlarged. With the availability of iodized salt, goiter has all but disappeared from this country. In other areas of the world, iodine deficiencies have been linked to mental retardation and breast cancer. Places where seafood or sea vegetable consumption is low and soil is iodine poor, iodine supplementation may be necessary.

Applications: thyroid health (goiter, hyperthyroidism), fibrocystic breast disease, endocrine system disorders

Daily Value: 150 micrograms

Optimal Consumption: For strict vegetarians who eat little salt and no seafood, 150 mcg per day is adequate.

Scientific Updates: A Canadian study found that supplemental iodine in three different forms improved fibrocystic breast disease in a group of test subjects. Over 70 percent of the women treated experienced improvement with molecular iodine obtaining the best results.

Depletors: salt-free diets and iodine-poor soil

Safety: Only small amounts of iodine are needed to help break down excess fat and contribute to thyroid health. Excess iodine can produce mouth sores, metallic taste, diarrhea, swollen salivary glands and possible vomiting. Keep in mind that iodine supplementation at levels greater than 3,000 mcg can result in a rebound goiter. Some people react to supplemental iodine with an acne-like rash.

Special Instructions: Look for iodine caseinate and kelp as good organic sources of iodine. Keep in mind that if you are using sea salt, it may not contain iodine.

Product Availability: Iodine supplements come as potassium iodine in tablet form. They are usually given to people on strict salt-free diets who may be prone to an iodine deficiency. You may also find iodine in the form of sodium iodide, protein-bound iodide and molecular iodine, which should only be used with the consent and supervision of your health care practitioner.

References

Ghent et al. 1993. Iodine replacement in fibrocystic disease of the breast. *Canadian Journal of Surgery* 36(5):453–60.

Iron

Overview: Iron is essential for the production of hemoglobin and red blood cell oxygenation. It is also essential for stamina, a healthy immune system, and the avoidance of anemia. Iron deficiency can cause pallor, hair loss, brittle nails, dizziness and anemia. Rheumatoid arthritis and cancer can contribute to iron depletion, causing anemia. Excessive menstrual bleeding, ulcer and poor digestion can also result in iron depletion. New studies point to iron as vital to maintaining a normal metabolism.

Daily Value: 18 milligrams

Optimal Consumption: A premenopausal woman who has periods can safely take up to 18 milligrams of iron daily. If you have been diagnosed with anemia, consult your doctor for higher dosages. All other people including children should not take supplemental iron unless advised to do so by a physician. Men are rarely iron deficient.

Scientific Updates: Iron deficiency anemia may contribute to faulty thyroid gland function, which could adversely affect metabolism. A recent study suggests that women with anemia may also fail to maintain normal metabolic rates, which could effect their energy levels and weight. Several other studies show that children who are anemic and take iron supplements actually improve their performance in school.

Depletors: blood loss, anemia, strict vegetarianism, pregnancy, heavy menstrual periods

Safety: Excess iron can produce free radicals and stomach upset. Children should not be given iron unless prescribed by physician for a particular disorder or malnutrition. Iron can be fatal to children if taken in an overdose. If you have heavy periods, have your iron levels checked before taking a supplement. Iron supplementation can cause constipation; and for anyone with hemochromatosis, taking iron supplements can be dangerous.

Special Instructions: Taking an excess of calcium, zinc or magnesium can interfere with the absorption of iron. Vitamin C enhances absorption. For optimal absorption, take iron on an empty stomach. As little as 25 milligrams of vitamin C can greatly enhance the absorption of iron. Avoid using enteric-coated or time-release capsules. Do not combine iron and calcium supplements or with antacids or high fiber foods. All of these decrease iron absorption. You may want to divide your doses over the day rather than taking an iron supplement all at once.

Product Availability: The most common and least expensive form of supplemental iron is ferrous sulfate. It is more prone to cause stomach upset, however. Iron fumarate and iron gluconate are less irritating, but can cause constipation.

References

Harris, Rosenzweig et al. 2000. Effect of iron supplementation on thyroid hormone levels and resting metabolic rate in two college female athletes: a case study. *International Journal of Sport Nutrition and Exercise Metabolism* 10(4):434-43.

Magnesium

Overview: Essential for calcium and potassium assimilation, magnesium contributes to proper nerve and muscle impulses and enzyme reactions. It plays a role in the formation of bone and in carbohydrate metabolism. New studies reveal its key role in muscle oxygenation especially during athletic activity. Magnesium is required to make ATP, which provides energy to our cells. It also acts as a natural antioxidant.

Daily Value: 400 milligrams

Optimal Consumption: Doses of magnesium over 400 milligrams should only be taken with the consent of your health care provider. Blood tests are available to determine whether you are magnesium deficient.

Applications: anxiety, asthma, depression, endometriosis, fibromyalgia, nervousness, muscle weakness, heart disease, dizziness, high blood pressure, PMS, heart arrhythmia, migraine headaches, angina, restless legs syndrome, Reynaud's disease, binge-eating disorder, osteoporosis, chronic fatigue syndrome, intermittent claudication, celiac disease, menstrual cramps, tinnitus, kidney stones, diabetes, insomnia, leg cramps

Scientific Updates: New studies show that women with fibromyalgia may not assimilate magnesium properly, thereby causing faulty muscle metabolism and subsequent pain. Most experts advise supplementation. Another study found that magnesium supplementation in test animals with hypertension significantly lowered their blood pressure.

Depletors: stress, diabetes, alcohol, diuretics, diarrhea, fluoride, digitalis, refined sugar and excess vitamin D

Safety: Check with your doctor before taking a magnesium supplement if you suffer from heart disease, heart arrhythmia, high blood pressure, migraine headaches, kidney disease, or if you are taking diuretic drugs. Diarrhea or frequent bowel movements can occur when magnesium is taken.

Special Instructions: If you take oxide and hydroxide forms of magnesium, you might have some diarrhea. Other forms of magnesium are thought to be more absorbable with less risk of diarrhea.

Product Availability: Magnesium is available in lactate, glycinate, orotate, gluconate, oxide and hydroxide forms. You may also find magnesium paired with calcium and vitamin D in bone formulas.

References

Kh et al. 2000. Effect of oral magnesium supplementation on blood pressure, platelet aggregation and calcium handling in deoxycorticosterone acetate induced hypertension in rats. *Journal of Hypertension* 8(7):919-26.

Ng, S.Y. 1999. Hair calcium and magnesium levels in patients with fibromyalgia: a case center study. *Journal of Manipulative Physiological Therapy* 2(9):586–93.

Manganese *(Trace mineral)*

Overview: Only tiny amounts of manganese are required for blood sugar regulation and fat and protein metabolism. Manganese is vital for proper bone growth and works in tandem with B-complex vitamins. It is needed for healthy skin, bone, and cartilage formation and also works to activate superoxide dismutase (SOD): a vital antioxidant enzyme.

Daily Value: 2 to 5 milligrams

Optimal Consumption: Many people fail to consume the daily value of manganese. People with osteoporosis or blood sugar disorders may need more and should consult their health care practitioner.

Applications: lactation, diabetes, hypoglycemia, asthma, muscle and mental fatigue, epilepsy, PMS, digestion, osteoporosis

Scientific Updates: New studies suggest that SOD may help to keep cells from replicating abnormally (what happens when cancer occurs).

Depletors: osteoporosis, nursing, diabetes, muscle fatigue

Safety: Dosages from 2 to 50 mg have not been associated with any toxicity. In rare cases, large doses of manganese may cause dementia and other psychiatric symptoms. If you have cirrhosis, you may not be able to excrete manganese, so you should avoid supplements.

Special Instructions: Antacids can interfere with manganese absorption as can excess magnesium, calcium, phosphorous and fiber. Too much manganese can also interfere with the assimilation of these same minerals. Copper and zinc work together with manganese to stimulate superoxide dismutase.

Product Availability: Manganese is usually contained in multiple formulas but can be purchased in picolinate or gluconate varieties.

References

Bernard et al. 2001. Antiproliferative and antiapoptotic effects of crel may occur within the same cells via the up-regulation of manganese superoxide dismutase. *Cancer Research* 15:61(6):2656–64.

Molybdenum *(trace mineral)*

Overview: Very tiny amounts of this essential mineral are needed for nitrogen metabolism. It also contributes to the metabolism of iron and in the detoxification of sulfites in the body. Low levels of molybdenum have been linked to mouth and gum disease, impotence and some cancers. It is also used to treat anemia.

Daily Value: 75 micrograms

Optimal Consumption: The estimated dosage range recommended for adults is between 75 and 250 mcg per day.

Applications: asthma, sulfite sensitivity, anemia, gingivitis, impotence

Scientific Updates: There is some scientific evidence that molybdenum supplementation inhibits the development of breast cancer.

Depletors: none known

Safety: Molybdenum is considered safe, but it can interfere with the absorption of copper. Molybdenum is also required to convert purine to uric acid. Therefore, large doses could cause gout-like symptoms, including joint pain or swelling. It should not be used in infants with phenylketonuria.

Special Instructions: New studies suggest that taking molybdenum with vitamin C may enhance its activity.

Product Availability: Molybdenum is often combined with other minerals in multiple formulas.

References

Seaborn, C. and S. Yang. 1993. Effect of molybdenum supplementation on N-nitroso- N-methylurea induced mammary carcinogenesis and molybdenum excretion in rats. *Biological Trace Elements Research* 39(2-3):245-56.

Phosphorus

Overview: Phosphorus is essential for bone and tooth development, heart muscle contraction and proper kidney health. It also contributes to the utilization of food for energy. It is one of the few nutrients we actually consume in excess. Carbonated beverages usually contain phosphorus. Calcium works with phosphorus to create crystal-like substances that give bone and teeth their strength. Excess phosphorus, however, can cause calcium to be poorly absorbed, resulting in bone weakness.

Daily Value: 1,000 milligrams

Optimal Consumption: Most of us need to reduce rather than enhance our phosphorus levels.

Applications: tooth and gum disease, sterility, impotence, equilibrium, muscle disorders, bone formation

Scientific Updates: The high consumption of carbonated beverages and the declining consumption of milk are of great concern for women because of their susceptibility to osteoporosis in later life.

Depletors: antacids containing aluminum

Safety: Taking excessive amounts of phosphorus can interfere with calcium absorption. The over consumption of carbonated beverages by young women can predispose them to osteoporosis.

Special Instructions: If phosphorus is taken in supplement form it must be balanced out with proper amounts of calcium. Vitamin D enhances the action of phosphorus. In rare cases, people who use antacids containing aluminum hydroxide may suffer from a phosphorus deficiency.

Product Availability: Because we have a tendency to take in too much phosphorus, supplementation is rare.

References

Wyshak, G. and R. Frisch. 1994. Carbonated beverages, dietary calcium, the dietary calcium/phosphorus ratio, and bone fractures in girls and boys. *Journal of Adolescent Health* 15(3):210-5.

Potassium

Overview: Potassium is an essential mineral that helps maintain the proper balance of cellular fluid with other electrolytes such as sodium and chloride, which in turn enables muscles to contract and relax. Potassium works in tandem with sodium for proper electrolyte balance. It contributes to heart muscle health, changes glycogen to glucose and promotes healing.

Daily Value: 3,500 milligrams

Optimal Consumption: Potassium depletion can occur during times of strenuous activity or excessive perspiration and must be replaced in electrolyte drinks, etc. No one should be taking a potassium supplement without the consent of his or her health care practitioner.

Applications: stress, times of exercise, diabetes, high blood pressure, stroke, leg cramps, heart arrhythmia, heat exhaustion.

Scientific Updates: Very recent studies suggest that potassium supplementation may help to increase endurance during periods of exercise.

Depletors: diuretics, excessive perspiration, steroids; alcohol, prolonged vomiting or diarrhea, overuse of laxatives, eating disorders.

Safety: Large doses of potassium are available only by prescription and should only be taken with medical supervision. Excessive potassium can disrupt the balance of other minerals and can also cause potentially fatal heart and kidney problems. People with kidney disease should not take it unless supervised by their physician. In addition, anyone taking digitalis, diuretics, and angiotensin-type hypertension drugs should not take potassium unless under the direct orders of their physician.

Special Instructions: Potassium/sodium ratios must be balanced in order for both to function properly. Too much sodium can disrupt the action of potassium and cause its excretion.

Product Availability: Potassium citrate or aspartate or any other chelated form is recommended. Potassium phosphate is also available.

References

Goss et al. 2001. Effect of potassium phosphate supplementation on perceptual and physiological responses to maximal graded exercise. *International Journal of Sports Nutrition and Exercise Metabolism* 11(1):53–62.

Selenium *(Trace Mineral)*

Overview: As an impressive antioxidant, selenium works well with vitamin E to scavenge free radicals, thus helping to prevent cellular mutation, cancers and the effects of aging. It also has significant anti-cancer actions and fights the spread of viral infections.

Daily Value: 70 micrograms

Optimal Consumption: Don't take selenium in doses over 200 micrograms daily without the supervision of your health care practitioner. Keep in mind that many drugs including chemotherapeutic agents can increase the body's selenium requirements.

Applications: cancer and cancer prevention, heart disease, immune dysfunction, angina, premature aging, cataracts, hair loss, chronic infections, viral infections, lupus, HIV, sexual dysfunction, menopause and skin ailments.

Scientific Updates: Taking selenium with beta-carotene significantly enhanced immune function in groups of test subjects. In addition, selenium has shown impressive anticancer activity.

Depletors: excess iron, malnutrition

Safety: Don't take more than 200 mcg in supplement form. High doses of selenium may cause brittle, thick nails, diarrhea, stomach cramps, numbness is the hands and feet, irritability and fatigue. Doses of 800 micrograms have caused tissue damage.

Special Instructions: If you are taking a single selenium supplement or as part of a combination formula, don't let your total selenium intake exceed 350 micrograms daily.

Product Availability: Selenium comes in selenomethionine and sodium selenite forms. Yeast supplements can also be high in selenium content.

References
Wood et al. 2000. Beta-carotene and selenium supplementation enhances immune response in aged humans. *Integrative Medicine* 21:2(2):85–92.

Silicon

Overview: Necessary for bone and collagen formation, silicon maintains the flexibility of arteries, counteracts the toxic effects of aluminum, and contributes to preventing cardiovascular disease. It may also play a role in the prevention of Alzheimer's disease by protecting the body from aluminum exposure. Silicon also helps maintain skin elasticity and may treat arthritis and other joint or cartilage problems. Silicon is also believed to contribute to the healing of fractures and may play a role in the prevention or treatment of osteoporosis.

Daily Value: none assigned

Optimal Consumption: A recommended intake of silicon has not been established. The average diet is estimated to provide 5 to 20 mg of silicon daily. When used in supplement form, doses range from 1 to 2 mg daily. Keep in mind that eating a diet high in processed foods and low in vegetables and grains can diminish silicon intake.

Applications: hair, skin, and nail health, tissue repair, aluminum protection, wrinkling, atherosclerosis, heart disease, arthritis, joint and cartilage problems, gastric ulcers, fractures, osteoporosis

Scientific Updates: New studies confirm the ability of silicon to reduce the accumulation of aluminum in tissue. If aluminum plays a role in Alzheimer's or Lou Gehrig's disease, silicon may afford some level of protection.

Depletors: poor nutrition

Safety: No known side effects. Considered non-toxic in recommended amounts. Inhalation of large amounts of silicon can cause a respiratory disease called silicosis.

Special Instructions: An herb called horsetail is a rich natural source of silicon. It is also sold as colloidal silicic acid and sodium metasilicate. To get extra silicon, eat more whole grains and fresh vegetables or use herbs such as alfalfa or horsetail.

Product Availability: Silicon is often found in herbal combinations designed to strengthen hair, skin and nails.

References

Belles et al. 1998. Silicon reduces aluminum accumulation in rats: relevance to the aluminum hypothesis of Alzheimer disease. *Alzheimer Dis Assoc Disord* 12(2):83–7.

Sodium

Overview: Essential for proper water and blood pH balance, stomach and nerve function, sodium can be lost during periods of excessive perspiration, vomiting or diarrhea. Inorganic sodium, which is found in table salt, can be detrimental if used in excess. Like phosphorus, our diets are usually too high in sodium which can, in some cases, contribute to water retention and high blood pressure.

Daily Value: 2,400 milligrams

Optimal Consumption: Like phosphorus, most of us need to reduce our sodium intake rather than boost it. The actual amount of sodium needed by the body to function properly is a source of significant controversy among doctors and scientists. Some discourage more than 500 milligrams daily while others suggest that amounts up to 5,000 milligrams are acceptable. One teaspoon of table salt contains about 2,000 milligrams of sodium. If your kidneys function properly, excess sodium will be excreted in the urine. Like phosphorus, if you have lost body fluids through excessive perspiration, diarrhea or vomiting, you may need to replace sodium in the form of an electrolyte beverage.

Applications: physical exertion, diarrhea, vomiting, excessive perspiration

Scientific Updates: While it is still accepted that sodium can aggravate high blood pressure, there is some speculation that sodium alone is not the only factor involved. Why eating a diet high in sodium causes some people to retain water and not others is still under investigation. It is still believed that most of us consume too much sodium.

Depletors: vomiting, excessive sweating, continual diarrhea, malnutrition

Safety: Taking too much sodium can result in water retention, hypertension, liver and kidney dysfunction and potassium depletion. In order to assimilate sodium properly, calcium, potassium, sulfur and vitamin D need to be present.

Special Instructions: Hidden sodium can be present in baking soda (sodium bicarbonate), monosodium glutamate (MSG), sodium propionate or any other ingredient prefaced by the word "sodium." Soft water also contains extra sodium.

Product Availability: Sodium chloride is the form found in common table salt.

References

Tikkanen et al. 1997. Delayed increase in blood pressure induced by spontaneously hypertensive rat plasma after high sodium intake. *Blood Pressure* 6(3):188–91.

Sulfur

Overview: Vital for cellular protection, sulfur has anti-aging properties and is needed for the formation of collagen. It also works to detoxify cells of harmful substances by bonding with them, thereby turning them into neutralized compounds that are excreted out of the body. Sulfur is absorbed from protein foods and water. Sulfur is not related to sulfa drugs or sulfites, which are found in some foods as preservative agents.

Daily Value: none assigned

Optimal Consumption: There is little concern about getting too much or too little sulfur.

Applications: blood purification, tissue repair, dandruff, acne, skin and hair strength, joint disease, irregular menstrual cycles

Scientific Updates: A new study suggests that people with gout suffer from sulfur accumulations that come from the consumption of protein foods and the creation of uric acid causing joint inflammation and pain. Sulfur may also be therapeutic in the treatment of arthritis and other inflammatory joint conditions.

Depletors: none known

Safety: Take as directed. Safe dosage ranges have not been established for this mineral. Sulfur can react with some prescription drugs and should not be taken as a single supplement under normal conditions. Don't take extra sulfur if you have gout. To be assimilated properly adequate amounts of vitamin B1, B5 and biotin need to be present.

Special Instructions: If you are using an amino acid formula as a source of sulfur, take it on an empty stomach with a little fruit juice.

Product Availability: One will rarely find a single sulfur supplement.

Sulfur is usually offered in amino acid supplements that contain cysteine, cystine, taurine or methionine. MSM (methylsulfonylmethane) is also considered a type of sulfur compound. Some individuals should reduce their sulfur intake.

References

Johnson, S. 1999. Effect of gradual accumulation of iron, molybdenum and sulfur, slow depletion of zinc and copper, ethanol or fructose ingestion and phlebotomy in gout. *Medical Hypotheses* 53(5):407–12.

Vanadium *(Trace Mineral)*

Overview: Required for good circulation and proper cholesterol levels, vanadium deficiencies have been linked to kidney and heart disease. Vanadium is difficult to absorb and deficiencies are linked to growth retardation, bone deformities and infertility. It may also play a role in building bones and teeth.

Daily Value: none assigned

Optimal Consumption: To date, vanadium supplementation is not usually advised. Optimal intake of vanadium remains unknown. It is estimated that the body's need for vanadium is probably less than 10 mcg per day. The average dietary intake is between 15 and 30 mcg per day.

Applications: goiter, diabetes, high cholesterol and heart disease.

Scientific Updates: Vanadyl sulfate, a form of vanadium may improve glucose control in people with non-insulin-dependent diabetes mellitus (NIDDM). According to a study of eight diabetics supplemented with 100 mg of the mineral daily for four weeks, vanadium lowered blood-sugar levels. The long-term safety of vanadium sulfate is not yet known.

Safety: Vanadium should not be taken in amounts over 100 mcg. If you are taking lithium, you should not use vanadium unless directed to do so by your physician. Vanadium has been shown to both inhibit and stimulate cancer growth in test animals.

Special Instructions: Vanadium should be taken in balance with other minerals and preferably not with chromium. Food processing and tobacco can interfere with the uptake of vanadium.

Product Availability: Vanadium is not easily absorbed and at this point, is not considered a single dietary supplement. It is usually found as vanadyl sulfate in nutritional supplement formulas.

References

Cusi et al. 2001. Vanadyl sulfate improves hepatic and muscle insulin sensitivity in type II diabetes. *Journal of Clinical Endocrinology Metabolism* 86(3):1410–7.

Zinc

Overview: The profound role of zinc in prostate gland disease is emerging. It is also essential for other reproductive organs and for strong immune function. Zinc is also involved in taste and smell and protects the liver from toxins.

Daily Value: 15 milligrams

Optimal Consumption: 18 mg daily is recommended for anyone who is taking extra calcium supplementation. Calcium interferes with zinc absorption.

Applications: prostate disease, infections, sterility, diabetes, wound healing and ulcers, kidney disease, diarrhea, liver disease, macular degeneration, cataracts, male infertility, hair loss, wound healing, impotence, dermatitis, canker sores, bedsores, loss of appetite, low immunity, taste and smell problems, genital herpes, binge-eating disorder, osteoarthritis, HIV, lupus, rheumatoid arthritis.

Scientific Updates: New studies suggest that zinc deficiencies can predispose individuals to lower immune response, thereby predisposing them to infections. Older individuals are particularly at risk.

Depletors: high-fiber foods, diabetes, alcohol, pregnancy, infection

Safety: Excessive doses of zinc can actually impair the immune system. Doses should be kept under 100 mg per day unless supervised by a physician. Zinc supplements can cause nausea if taken on an empty stomach, and zinc lozenges can dry out the mouth.

Special Instructions: Calcium, iron and often high-fiber diets interfere with zinc absorption. Large amounts of zinc impair copper absorption. Taking 20 mg a day of zinc is customary.

Product Availability: Zinc picolinate, acetate, citrate, and monomethionine are recommended. Zinc throat lozenges may help treat colds.

References

Fortes et al. 1998. The effect of zinc and vitamin A supplementation on immune response in an older population. *Journal of American Geriatric Society* 46(1):19–26.

Amino Acids & Antioxidants

Amino acids are the building blocks of proteins and are vital to life. For a protein to be considered a whole unit, it must contain a complete amino acid array. Linking different amino acids together can create over 50,000 types of proteins and 20,000 known enzymes. Each protein has its specific amino acid signature. Approximately twenty commonly known amino acids exist. The liver produces 80 percent of the amino acids we need to sustain life. The remaining 20 percent must be obtained from the diet and are therefore referred to as essential amino acids. Amino acids enable vitamins and minerals to act properly within our biosystems. If any of these amino acids are missing, the assimilation and utilization of these other nutrients will be impaired. Today, amino acid therapy is emerging as an exciting source of therapeutic treatment. Recent studies confirm that certain amino acids when taken singly or in combination can exert the same types of medicinal effects as some prescription drugs.

Amino Acid Deficiencies Can Occur

Once again, the common assumption may be that the majority of Americans get plenty of amino acids in their diets, which are typically high in meat and eggs. Ironically, the opposite may actually be the case. Diets that are not balanced and are high on empty carbohydrates can become protein deficient. Balance is the key. Even though we are well aware of the perils of a diet that is too high in protein, most of us do not eat high-quality protein foods. Red meat is not the only source of protein and amino acids. Other protein foods including nuts, beans, soy products, fish and eggs, which are excellent sources of protein. Unfortunately the majority of people eat diets that are deficient in the total amino acid array we need to maintain our health.

Commercial Amino Acid Preparations

Amino acid supplements are available in single or combination form and are often part of a complete multivitamin or protein supplement formula. They come in capsules, powders, or tablets and are usually derived from soy, egg or yeast protein. The term "crystalline free form" refers to amino acids extracted from grain sources such as brown rice bran. Free-form amino acids are recommended in that they are rapidly assimilated. Amino acids are best taken on an empty stomach with a little fruit juice. If you take them with protein foods, their absorption can be compromised. Generally speaking, taking specific amino acids for individual disorders is more effective than just using supplemental combinations of amino acids.

Safety Concerns

Don't take amino acid supplements without your doctor's approval. Although amino acids are generally considered safe, their long-term effects on health remain unknown. We do know that large doses of arginine may cause nausea and diarrhea. If you have genital herpes, you should avoid arginine. Arginine and lysine should not be taken together or both of their actions may be compromised. Cysteine in high doses may cause kidney stones if you have a condition called cystinuria. It can also decrease the action of insulin. If you have diabetes, only use cysteine with your doctor's supervision. Cysteine supplementation may also deplete the body of zinc and copper. Tyrosine and phenylalanine supplements may substantially raise blood pressure, especially in people taking MAO inhibitors as antidepressants. You should not take supplemental phenylalanine if you have phenylketonuria.

Therapeutic Applications of Amino Acids

depression, heart disease, high blood pressure, low immunity, indigestion, heartburn, diarrhea, obesity, diverticulitis, prostate problems, intermittent claudication, infertility, tissue repair, muscle building

Note: Alanine, glutamic acid and glycine taken together may relieve the symptoms of benign prostatic hyperplasia(BPH).

Single Amino Acids and Their Physiological Actions

L-Alanine: Involved in the metabolism of glucose and recommended for hypoglycemia

L-Arginine*: Retards tumor growth, increases sperm count and promotes the formation of lean muscle mass and the proper formation of scar tissue. Do not take if pregnant or lactating

L-Asparagine: Nourishes the central nervous system, promoting emotional stability

L-Aspartic Acid: Boosts energy and endurance by enhancing liver toxin removal

L-Carnitine: Prevents fatty buildup and boosts fatty acid utilization

L-Citrulline: Promotes energy and detoxifies ammonia from cells

L-Cysteine: Detoxifies cells and is an excellent free radical scavenger that also promotes muscle mass

L-Cystine: Protects against copper toxicity, promotes healing and contributes to insulin formation

Gamma-Amino butyric Acid: Considered a natural tranquilizer, it decreases neuron activity

L-Glutamic Acid: Metabolizes sugars and fats and helps fight brain and mental disorders

L-Glutamine: Good for treating alcoholism, sugar cravings, epilepsy, mental disorders and ulcers

L-Glutathione: A powerful antioxidant that protects against radiation, smoke, x-rays and alcohol

L-Glycine: Used for bipolar depression, prostate gland, and central nervous system health

L-Histidine*: Repairs tissue and is good for rheumatoid arthritis, anemia and allergies

L-Isoleucine*: Essential for hemoglobin formation, regulates blood sugar and energy levels

L-Leucine*: Decreases blood sugar and boosts tissue healing including bone. Recommended for post-surgery convalescence. An excess of this amino acid can cause hypoglycemia

L-Lysine*: Inhibits virus infections and is recommended for Herpes simplex, cankers, cold sores

L-Methionine*: Breaks down fats and detoxifies tissue, assists with choline production

L-Ornithine: When combined with carnitine and arginine, breaks down excess body fat

L-Phenylalanine*: Needed to make neurotransmitters, aids in depression, memory and migraines. Can also act as an appetite suppressant

DL-Phenylalanine: Suppresses appetite and helps control arthritic pain. Do not use if pregnant or if you have high blood pressure or diabetes

L-Proline: Contributes to the production of collagen, strengthens joints and tendons

L-Serine: Contributes to strong immune functions and helps your body metabolize fats and promote muscle mass

L-Taurine: A key component of bile, good for cholesterol levels, hyperactivity, epilepsy and brain function

L-Threonine*: Helps control epilepsy and aids in formation of elastin and collagen

L-Tryptophan*: Contributes to serotonin production, stabilizes moods, promotes sleep and stress control. **Note:** In 1989: all tryptophan was taken off the market due to a batch contaminated with EMS, a blood disorder. The FDA has recalled all products containing tryptophan; however, new modified forms of tryptophan such as 5HTP (5-hydroxy-tryptophan)are available

L-Tyrosine: Important for brain function and can help with depression, headaches, anxiety and food cravings

L-Valine*: Acts as a natural stimulant and is involved in tissue regeneration and nitrogen balance

*Amino acids that are considered essential and that must be obtained from the diet.

Amino Acid Products: Recommendations

Amino acid preparations are readily available at health food stores in the form of capsules, powders and liquids. Their sources are usually animal, yeast or vegetable proteins. Brown rice, milk protein and yeast sources are viable sources. More companies are offering amino acid supplements. Some simple guidelines to follow are as follows:

1. Look for USP (U.S. Pharmacopoeia) or pharmaceutical grade products that are denoted by the letter L and by the word crystalline. *Note:* Phenylalanine comes in the DL form.
2. Look for free form products, which are much easier to digest and assimilate and are considered less allergenic. Capsulized powdered forms are best.
3. Take amino acids on an empty stomach with a little fruit juice. If you take them with meals, the other nutrients you have ingested will compete with the amino acids for absorption. Make sure that you will not be eating for at least thirty minutes before or after taking an amino acid supplement.
4. Amino acid therapy should be short term, rather than indefinite. Large doses are discouraged. Taking a break from supplementation is also recommended; i.e., two months on, two months off. Children should not be given amino acid supplements unless under the supervision of a physician.

Antioxidants

Twentieth-century life exposes us to a whole host of new and potentially harmful toxins. Virtually every day most of us encounter countless pollutants, which cause the formation of damaging oxidants in our bodies. Auto exhaust, tobacco smoke, UV rays, pollution, preservatives, food additives and chemicals used to purify our water continually assault our biocellular systems. As a result, our risk of developing a degenerative disease is significantly increased. Moreover, our constant exposure to these oxidizing agents can accelerate premature tissue breakdown causing us to age more rapidly. Inevitably, regardless of where or how we live, we will find ourselves impacted by substances that break down our cellular structures.

Though this declaration sounds ominous, at best, Mother Nature has provided us with some very impressive defense compounds called antioxidants. These remarkable nutrients have the capability to protect us from the perils of oxidants or free radicals as they are also called. Even though common sense measures such as eating nutritiously and living a healthy lifestyle should be our first line of defense, we need extra fortification.

Free Radicals

A free radical is nothing more than a molecular structure that contains an unpaired electron. Electrons like to co-exist in pairs. Electron couples make up the chemical bond that keeps molecules from flying apart. An unpaired electron is driven by a potent chemical force that compels it to find a mate. This molecular instinct to merge with another electron is so powerful that the searching molecule behaves erratically, moving about much like a weapon within cellular structures. Its random and wild molecular movements within cellular material can create cellular damage, which eventually results in degeneration or mutation.

Why Are Free Radicals So Dangerous?

A free radical can destroy a protein, an enzyme, or even a complete cell. To make matters worse, free radicals can multiply through a chain reaction mechanism resulting in the release of thousands of these cellular oxidants. When this happens, cells can become so badly damaged that DNA codes can be altered and immunity can be compromised. In some cases, abnormal cellular growth in the form of tumors can result. Contact with free radicals on this scale can create cellular deterioration, resulting in diseases like cancer. Tissue breakdown from this oxidative stress can also occur, contributing to aging, arthritis and whole host of other degenerative conditions. Constant free radical bombardment has been compared to being irradiated at low levels all of the time.

Free radical damage has been associated with over sixty known diseases and disorders. Some of the more dangerous free radical producing substances include the following:

cigarette smoke
herbicides
pesticides
smog
car exhaust
certain prescription drugs
diagnostic and therapeutic x-rays
ultra-violet light
gamma radiation
rancid foods
certain fats
alcohol
some of our food and water supplies
stress

Even exercising, as beneficial as it is, can initiate the release of free radicals within our cellular systems. Aerobic exercising produces damaging oxidation byproducts. Many of these are not completely neutralized by internal safety mechanisms, and an overload can occur. Supplementing the diet with effective antioxidant compounds is highly recommended for everyone, especially for those who exercise regularly.

Cigarette Smoke

When cigarette smoke is inhaled in the lungs, billions of free radicals are subsequently released into the blood stream. Even passive smokers who are only exposed to second hand smoke experience this surge of oxidants. Smokers are at high risk for developing heart disease and cancer. It is thought that by increasing antioxidant supplementation, smokers can help to lessen free radical damage, and as a result, decrease their disease risk.

Alcohol

Consuming certain amounts of alcohol can also produce free radicals in the liver, which can eventually lead to cirrhosis, heart disease and cancer. In his book, *Natural Health, Natural Medicine*, Andrew Weil, M.D. states "Heavy drinkers are at greater risk of developing cancers of the mouth, throat, esophagus and stomach, probably because alcohol irritates those tissues directly. Heavy drinkers are also more likely to get liver cancer. The danger is compounded if you also smoke tobacco."

Air Pollution

Heavily polluted areas such as smoggy cities can create what is called an oxidant ozone, which results in cellular damage related to free radical injury. Congested metropolitan areas have notoriously high levels of carbon monoxide. Industries continually pump harmful particulates into our air supply, not to mention a number of caustic chemicals.

High-Fat, High-Protein Diets

While certain fats are bad for us, others can be very health promoting when consumed in moderation. Hydrogenated fats should be avoided if possible. These fats contain trans-fatty acids, which tend to clog arteries and produce free radical tissue damage. Even an excess of polyunsaturated fats can pose health dangers in the form of free radicals. The process used to harden polyunsaturates into products like margarine creates these harmful acids, which can contribute to cardiovascular disease. It is the process of oxidation that is so potentially harmful to all of us. Using monounsaturated fats like olive oil is highly recommended. Essential fatty acids supplements are also beneficial.

Free Radicals and Cancer

Numerous research studies support the fact that many cancers (breast cancer in particular) are diet related. Moreover, the risks of certain kinds of cancer can be significantly reduced with dietary changes. While most of us are aware of the wonders of a low-fat diet, a tremendous amount of data conceding other cancer-preventative nutrients never reaches the average consumer. For example, recent studies suggest that just reducing dietary fat may not be enough to prevent certain cancers. In light of this notion, perhaps research should focus on why some cultures that eat fat still have low cancer rates? Perhaps it's not so much a question of what we eat, but what we don't eat. More and more research suggests that it is a lack of certain protective nutrients that appear to originate from dietary sources that increase our risk of cancer and other degenerative diseases. Taking the best of the antioxidants is one of the wisest moves we can make.

Antioxidants: Nature's Best Defense against Free Radicals

It has now been established that more than sixty human diseases involve free-radical damage, including cancer and heart disease. Several natural protectants against free radicals, which are also called free radical scavengers, have the chemical ability to donate electrons to free radical molecules, thereby making them more stable and less dangerous. Some of the most common of these free radical scavengers or antioxidants include:

vitamin E
vitamin C
vitamin A and beta-carotene
coenzyme Q10
selenium
proanthocyanidins (grapeseed or pinebark extracts)
glutathione
alpha-lipoic acid
superoxide dismutase
bioflavonoids
melatonin
bilberry (herb)
ginkgo (herb)

Note: I discuss each of the antioxidant compounds listed in more detail in the appropriate reference sections of this book.

Bioflavonoids

Bioflavonoids are another class of antioxidant nutrients. Bioflavonoids include the following: quercitin, rutin, hesperidin, naringin, indole-3-carbinol, proanthocyanidins and others. The term bioflavonoid refers to a large family of chemicals found throughout the plant world. Bioflavonoids are sometimes called vitamin P; however, they are not technically vitamins. So what exactly is a bioflavonoid? Bioflavonoids are phytochemicals or plant derivatives that can have remarkable effects on biochemical pathways in human physiology. There are over 20,000 known bioflavonoids registered in chemical abstracts, and over twenty million structures that fit into their chemical classification. Obviously not all flavonoids are the same.

For this reason, selecting the most biologically valuable compounds is extremely important when designing any supplement that utilizes bioflavonoid compounds. Bioflavonoids occur naturally in fruits and vegetables but they are subject to rapid decomposition and degradation during storage and cooking. Bioflavonoids are considered synergists to vitamin C and must be combined with vitamin C (ascorbic acid) for optimal benefit.

Bioflavonoids are among some of nature's most protective phytochemicals and work to protect the integrity of cell structures. They also work to strengthen capillaries, enhance connective tissue repair, decrease the risk of heart disease and stroke, and help prevent cancer.

Naringen, Hesperitin and Rutin

These three bioflavonoids are powerful antioxidants and work synergistically with vitamin C and the proanthocyanidins to scavenge free radicals. Moreover, this particular trio of flavonoids has significant antiallergenic properties. Studies have indicated that these compounds can inhibit the release of histamine, the chemical that causes a whole host of miserable allergic symptoms. Several laboratory tests support the fact that these flavonoids can significantly decrease inflammation by preventing histamine from permeating vessel walls. Obviously, any allergic condition, edema or other inflammatory diseases would substantially benefit from this vascular action. In addition, if you bruise easily, this group of bioflavonoids is particularly desirable. Naringin and hesperitin prevent capillary fragility and interstitial bleeding.

Quercetin

Quercitin is another remarkable flavonoid. Its particular antioxidant activity has been found to help reduce the risk of coronary heart disease. Quercitin helps dilate and relax blood vessels and has a protective effect against certain types of heart arrhythmia. It is the major active component of ginkgo biloba and may be responsible for the beneficial effects that ginkgo has on brain neurons. Quercitin has also shown antitumor properties. Its antiviral activity is particularly significant today, as we face new viral diseases capable of adjusting to various pharmacological treatments. Quercitin helps to protect the body against viral or bacterial invasion if given before an infection progresses. It may also help to prevent asthmatic symptoms.

Seven Chinese herbal drugs were screened for their ability to inhibit enzymes that cause several complications associated with diabetes. Quercitin was among the compounds tested and exhibited a potent action against these destructive enzymes. Anyone who suffers from diabetes should be aware of the potential benefit of quercitin.

Quercitin was also able to help normalize hormone levels in both males and females. The effect that quercitin demonstrated on female estrogen and male testosterone levels suggests that the flavonoid is valuable in treating women with high estrogen-related problems and men who suffer from prostate disorders. While quercitin has not been clinically tested for its ability to treat migraine headaches, its activity as a mast cell stabilizer suggests that it may be useful.

Bioflavonoid Applications

Ailmens and health conditions for which bioflavonoids may be useful include: allergies, asthma, carpal tunnel syndrome, bruises, gout, high cholesterol, varicose veins, hemorrhoids, low immunity, arthritis, and sciatica; with vitamin C, used for gingivitis, colds and flu, canker sores, cold sores, menopausal discomforts, heavy menstrual bleeding, vaginitis, and genital herpes.

How To Use Antioxidants

Taking a broad spectrum antioxidant is the best way to go. Why? Because we know that antioxidants work in the body at different sites. A person needs a good variety of free radical scavengers in both vitamin and herb form. Look for formulas that at minimum contain bioflavonoids, vitamin E, vitamin C and beta-carotene.

Nutritional Supplements

Acidophilus (see Probiotics)

Bee Pollen

Definition: Bee pollen is a fine powdery substance collected and stored by honeybees from the stamen found within a flower blossom. Experts consider bee pollen a highly nutritious, complete food. It contains a rich supply of B-complex vitamins, vitamins C, A, E, carotenoids, folic acid, amino acids, a wide array of minerals and some essential fatty acids.

Recommended for: allergies, asthma, impotence, indigestion, infections, sore throat, acne, fatigue, prostate disease

Scientific Updates: A new study has confirmed the antimicrobial action of bee pollen against certain strains of strep bacteria. People have used it for generations to promote stamina and restore energy after debilitating conditions. Although studies are lacking, herbalists promote it as a prostate protector.

Safety: If you suffer from pollen allergies, be judicious when taking bee pollen. Take granulized supplements with meals, and begin with small doses, working up to a teaspoon if you have had no adverse reaction. Once you have established that you tolerate the granules, you can then take bee pollen in other supplemental forms including tablets, powders, liquids, etc. Freeze-dried products are also available, and if possible request pollen from local bees. Do not take bee pollen if you have a history of anaphylactic reactions. Allergic reactions range from itching in the mouth and throat, to stomach pain to asthma attacks. If you have asthma or diabetes, don't take bee pollen unless approved by your doctor.

Product Forms: You can purchase bee pollen as a fresh powder, granules, chewable wafers, capsulized or in tablet form. It is also available in ointments and creams.

Comments: Purchase a supplement designed for internal use from a reliable source (to avoid contamination), and keep it refrigerated. The nutrient content of bee pollen is highly perishable.

References
Greenberger, P. and M. Flais. 2001. Bee pollen-induced anaphylactic reaction in an unknowingly sensitized subject. *Ann Allergy Asthma Immunol* 86(2):239–42.

Tichy, J. and J. Novak. 2000. Detection of antimicrobials in bee products with activity against viridans streptococci. *J Altern Complement Med* 6(5):383–9.

Bee Propolis

Definition: Bee propolis is a resinous substance that honeybees gather from deciduous tree bark and leaves. It is a sticky material that bees efficiently use to seal hive holes or cracks. Before they use it in the hive, honeybees take the sap and combine it with nectar found in their own secretions. Bees must transform resin into propolis, and only they know how. Propolis has been used for millennia as a protection against infection, a promoter of healing, and as a superior source of energy and endurance.

Recommended for: allergies, bruises, burns, cancer, dental hypersensitivity, herpes zoster, fatigue, sore throats, respiratory ailments, acne, sunburn, shingles

Scientific Updates: A new study found that bee propolis was able to successfully treat 85 percent of test subjects suffering from dentinal hypersensitivity.

Safety: Experts generally considered bee propolis to be safe, but like bee pollen, you should initially take it in small amounts to check for potential allergic reactions. Do not take bee propolis if you have asthma or are prone to allergic rashes or anaphylactic shock.

Product Forms: You can purchase bee propolis in tablets, cough syrups, toothpaste, mouthwash, skin lotions, throat sprays, ointments and tinctures.

Comments: Always buy bee products from established manufacturers that guarantee the purity of their products. Take propolis with food, and keep it refrigerated.

References
Mahmoud et al. 1999. The effect of propolis on dentinal hypersensitivity and level of satisfaction among patients from a university hospital Riyadh, Saudi Arabia. *Indian J Dent Res* 10(4):130–7.

Bioflavonoids

(The bioflavonoid family includes daflon, diosmetin, diosmin, hesperidin, naringin, narirutin, neohesperidin, nobiletin, rutin, tangeretin)

Definition: Bioflavonoids (also called *flavonoids*) comprise a group of plant pigments, which provide excellent cellular protection by modifying the action of allergens, carcinogens and viruses. Flavonoids are responsible for giving plants and their blossoms color pigment and are also found in the white material located just beneath the peel of citrus fruits. Although they are not technically vitamins, bioflavonoids are sometimes referred to as vitamin P. These remarkable free radical scavengers have many diverse health benefits especially for blood vessel integrity. Because the body cannot produce bioflavonoids, they must be supplied through diet or supplementation.

Recommended for: bruising, bleeding (including heavy menstrual flow), high cholesterol, cataracts, oral herpes, hemorrhoids, nosebleeds, swelling, varicose veins, allergies, asthma, liver disease, gum disease, diabetes, post-mastectomy lymph swelling

Scientific Updates: Several recent studies confirm the use of bioflavonoids for hemorrhoids, compromised circulation in the legs and accompanying leg ulcers, and for people who bruise easily or are prone to nosebleeds. The ability of bioflavonoids to inhibit swelling is of particular value for the lymphedema that often occurs after breast cancer surgery. Bioflavonoids also act as natural anti-inflammatory agents, may reduce cholesterol levels, and may even protect against cancer.

Safety: Excessively high doses may cause diarrhea. Diosmin and hesperidin have been designated as nontoxic even for pregnant women and small children. An overall increase in citrus bioflavonoids in the diet of pregnant women as been linked to the possibility of infant leukemia. Tangeretin may interfere with the action of tamoxifen, a drug used to treat breast cancer.

Product Forms: Bioflavonoids are usually combined with other vitamins, such as vitamin C, and are generally taken in capsule or tablet from. Some citrus derived powders that can be mixed with liquid are also available.

Comments: A typical dose of bioflavonoids is 500 mg taken twice daily. If you have been bruised or have a condition that causes significant swelling, you may want to increase that dose. Check with your doctor. Vitamin C often comes with various bioflavonoids.

References

Bracke et al. 1999. Influence of tangeretin on tamoxifen's therapeutic benefit in mammary cancer. J Natl Cancer Inst 91:354–359.

Guilhou et al. 1997. Efficacy of Daflon 500 mg in venous leg ulcer healing: a double-blind, randomized, controlled versus placebo trial in 107 patients. *Angiology* 48:77–85.

Misra, M. and R. Parshad. 2000. Randomized clinical trial of micronized flavonoids in the early control of bleeding from acute internal haemorrhoids. *Br J Surg* 87:868–872.

Pecking et al. 1997. Efficacy of Daflon 500 mg in the treatment of lymphedema (secondary to conventional therapy of breast cancer). *Angiology* 48:93–98.

Shin et al. 1999. Hypocholesterolemic effect of naringin associated with hepatic cholesterol regulating enzyme changes in rats. *Int J Vitam Nutr Res* 69:341–347.

So et al. 1996. Inhibition of human breast cancer cell proliferation and delay of mammary tumorigenesis by flavonoids and citrus juices. *Nutr Cancer* 26:167–181.

Strick et al. 2000. Dietary bioflavonoids induce cleavage in the MLL gene and may contribute to infant leukemia. *Proc Natl Acad Sci* 97:4790–4795.

Bovine Cartilage

Definition: Bovine cartilage is a tough, rubbery tissue that is extracted primarily from the windpipes of cows. Sharks and other animals can also provide cartilage sources. This tough material is what cushions our joints. It contains calcium, protein substances, collagen and carbohydrate mucopolysaccharides, which include a substance called chondroitin. Recently, the use of cartilage supplements has gained notoriety for arthritis and for some types of cancerous tumors. It has natural anti-inflammatory properties and can also decrease pain.

Recommended for: osteoarthritis, rheumatoid arthritis, joint injuries, pancreatic, liver and kidney tumors, fibromyalgia

Scientific Updates: Recent studies have found that bovine cartilage supplementation may help to shrink cancerous tumors in the kidney. Bovine cartilage contains substances that may block the growth of new blood vessels that nourish tumors, thereby depriving them of oxygen. This action has not been confirmed in oral supplementation. It is also thought that bovine cartilage boosts immune defenses against cancer cells. Bovine cartilage supplements may also help to stimulate matrix production of cartilage in damaged joints.

Product Forms: You can buy bovine cartilage in 750 mg capsules. It is often added to joint support formulas.

Safety: Mild stomach upset, nausea or fatigue can occur with supplementation. Pregnant or nursing women, children, or anyone with heart or vascular disease should not use cartilage products. You should not use cartilage products if you have recently had surgery or sustained a major injury because it may interfere with the regeneration of new blood vessels.

Comments: If you want a joint disease treatment, look for a comprehensive formula, including bovine cartilage, glucosamine and chondroitin products.

References

Puccio et al. 1994. Treatment of metastatic renal cell carcinoma with Catrix. *Proc Annu Meet Am Soc Clin Oncol* 13:A769

Wojtowicz-Praga, S. 1999. Clinical potential of matrix metalloprotease inhibitors. *Drugs R D (New Zealand)* 1:117–129.

Bovine Colostrum

Definition: Colostrum is the fluid produced in the breasts 24 to 48 hours after birth. It is rich in nutrients and immune factors like antibodies which afford protection to the newborn. Bovine colostrum comes from the cow and is a relatively new supplement. Bovine colostrum contains several compounds that can benefit the gastrointestinal tract and boost immunity.

Recommended for: immune dysfunction or weakness, infectious diarrhea, chronic infections, colitis or irritable bowel syndrome, mouth sores, Crohn's disease, stamina

Scientific Updates: Studies suggest that colostrum may benefit infectious diarrhea although most tests do not use bovine colostrum. Hyperimmune colostrum refers to colostrum from cows that have been immunized against certain diseases. Colostrum may also be good for bowel syndrome (a condition following digestive tract surgery) and chemotherapy-induced mouth ulcers. A new study shows that it helps to inhibit inflammatory stomach and colon conditions. Colostrum may also treat *Cryptosporidium* infection in people suffering from AIDS, shigella, and *E. coli*. It may also help to strengthen the immune system.

Safety: Colostrum appears to be safe, although it may cause an allergic reaction in individuals sensitive to milk products or immunoglobulins. Studies have not established its safety in young children or women who are pregnant or nursing.

Product Availability: Colostrum is now available in capsules as a dry powder. It may also be included in other products designed to treat bowel disorders or immune dysfunction.

Comments: The usual dosage of bovine colostrum is 10 g daily.

References

Antonio et al. 2001. The effects of bovine colostrum supplementation on body composition and exercise performance in active men and women. *Nutrition Mar* 17(3):243–7.

Graczyk et al. 2000. Successful hyperimmune bovine colostrum treatment of Savanna monitors (Varanus exanthematicus) infected with Cryptosporidium. *J Parasitol* 86(3):631–2.

Greenberg et al. 1996. Treatment of severe diarrhea caused by Cryptosporidium parvum with oral bovine immunoglobulin concentrate in patients with AIDS. *J Acquir Immune Defic Syndr Hum Retrovirol* 13:348–354.

Pacyna et al. 2001. Survival of rotavirus antibody activity derived from bovine colostrum after passage through the human gastrointestinal tract. *J Pediatr Gastroenterol Nutr* 32(2):162–7.

Playford et al. 2001. Co-administration of the health food supplement, bovine colostrum, reduces the acute non-steroidal anti-inflammatory drug-induced increase in intestinal permeability. *Clin Sci* 100(6):627–33.

Sugisawa et al. 2001. Promoting effect of colostrum on the phagocytic activity of bovine polymorphonuclear leukocytes in vitro. *Biol Neonate* 79(2):140–4.

Tacket et al. 1992. Efficacy of bovine milk immunoglobulin concentrate in preventing illness after Shigella flexneri challenge. *Am J Trop Med Hyg* 47:276–283.

Brewer's Yeast

Definition: Designated yeasts include baker's, brewer's and nutritional yeast. Most of us are familiar with the living yeast that makes baked goods rise. The living cells found in brewer's yeast offers a rich array of B-vitamins and minerals. Nutritional yeast refers to yeast cultivated with vitamin B12 and other nutrient compounds. You can find customized yeast that contains high levels of chromium or other minerals.

Recommended for: diabetes, eczema, restless leg syndrome, hypoglycemia, high cholesterol, nervousness, fatigue, constipation, boils, staph infections, strict vegans

Safety: Do not take Brewer's yeast if you are allergic to molds, have diabetes, hypoglycemia, yeast infections and gout. It may cause intestinal gas or digestive upset if taken on an empty stomach.

Scientific Updates: As a rich source of chromium, brewer's yeast has been used in blood sugar disorders. Chromium acts with insulin to transfer blood sugar through cell membranes to be used for energy. In addition, the chromium found in this supplement may also help to raise good cholesterol (HDL) while lowering the bad kind (LDL).

Product Forms: Brewer's yeast is available in powders, chewable tablets, flakes and capsules.

Comments: Because Brewer's yeast has a strong smell and taste, taking tablets may be more appealing, especially for younger individuals.

References

Bahijiri et al. The effects of inorganic chromium and brewer's yeast supplementation on glucose tolerance, serum lipids and drug dosage in individuals with type 2 diabetes. *Saudi Med Journal* 21(9)2000:831–837.

Bromelain

Definition: Bromelain is actually a combination of enzymes that exist in the pineapple fruit and its stem. We refer to these enzymes as "proteolytic," or having the ability to digest protein. Bromelain is commonly added into digestive enzyme formulas designed to boost digestion of milk, meat, eggs, fish, etc. and are also used in products that tenderize meats. In addition, bromelain helps to reduce swelling and bruising by breaking down substances called fibrins and kinins, which cause inflammation.

Recommended for: indigestion, diarrhea, muscle strains and sprains, colitis, bruising, wounds, post-surgery, arthritis, gout, bronchitis, urinary tract infections, varicose veins, insect bites, geriatric nutrition

Scientific Updates: A new trial found that using bromelain and other enzymes boosted the utilization of protein in older nursing home patients. Another study suggests that bromelain may benefit people suffering with rheumatoid arthritis. A significant number of test subjects found relief after thirteen weeks of treatment with no side effects. Other studies point to its ability to boost immune function and to treat diarrhea. It has also proven its ability to reduce swelling and pain after tissue injury and may benefit people with mild cases of colitis.

Product Forms: You can buy bromelain in chewable tablets and capsules. Experts recommend enteric forms for arthritis and other inflammatory conditions because enteric forms do not break down in the stomach. Common doses range between 250 and 1,000 mg.

Safety: Bromelain is considered nontoxic but can cause allergic reactions in certain sensitive individuals. Do not combine it with blood thinning drugs.

Comments: Apply pastes of bromelain (made by mixing the powder with a little water or witch hazel) as poultices for insect bites, bee stings, bruises and muscle injuries. It can also be taken internally as well.

References

Glade et al. 2001. Improvement in protein utilization in nursing-home patients on tube feeding supplemented with an enzyme product derived from Aspergillus niger and Bromelain. *Nutrition* 7(4):348–50.

Kane, S. and M. Goldberg. 2000. Use of bromelain for mild ulcerative colitis. *Ann Intern Med* 18:132(8):680.

Masson, M. 1995. Bromelain in blunt injuries of the locomotor system. A study of observed applications in general practice. *Fortschr Med* 113(19):303–06.

Mynott et al. 1997. Bromelain prevents secretion caused by Vibrio cholerae and Escherichia coli enterotoxins in rabbit ileum in vitro. *Gastroenterology* 113(1):175–84.

Netti et al. 1972. Anti-inflammatory action of proteolytic enzymes of animal vegetable or bacterial origin administered orally compared with that of known anti-phlogistic compounds. *Farmaco [Prat]* 27(8):453–66.

Chitosan

Definition: Chitosan is a fiber-like natural product made from the exoskeleton of shellfish; i.e., lobsters, crabs and shrimp. It is not digestible and has the ability to absorb many times its weight in fat, thereby preventing fat absorption through the intestinal walls and decreasing fecal transit time. Recently, it has generated a great deal of publicity as part of several weight-loss supplements, some of which have rather sensational claims.

Recommended for: obesity, high cholesterol, hypertension, heartburn, gout

Scientific Updates: Most studies on chitosan have been done with laboratory animals, and some do support its ability to inhibit fat absorption. In both rats and chicken, chitosan appeared to block the absorption of dietary fat. Initial results on human studies have had mixed reviews. Some have reported modest weight losses, and others have not. The general consensus is that if taken in the right amounts and at the right time, chitosan may inhibit the absorption of some dietary fat. Other studies suggest that it lowers blood cholesterol levels.

Safety: Children, pregnant or nursing women, or people with allergies to shellfish should not use chitosan. It can also block the absorption of fat-soluble vitamins and fatty acids and may cause loose stools or intestinal distress. Drinking 6 to 8 glasses of water daily helps to avoid possible intestinal obstruction. Chitosan may bind with certain medications thereby reducing their potency.

Product Availability: Stores sell chitosan in capsules and in powdered form that you can add to weight-loss formulas that contain other compounds. Taking vitamin C with chitosan may enhance its action.

Comments: It is best to take a full 8-ounce glass of water with each dose of chitosan to keep the bowels moving. Take a chitosan supplement thirty minutes prior to each meal. Keep in mind that it only works on meals containing fat. Do not take your vitamins or other supplements at the same time as chitosan. You will probably need 3 to 5 grams of chitosan with each meal to achieve optimal fat binding. Chances are that taking chitosan without changing your diet or exercise regimen will not achieve desired weight loss.

References

Chiang et al. 2000. Effect of dietary chitosans with different viscosity on plasma lipids and lipid peroxidation in rats fed on a diet enriched with cholesterol. *Biosci Biotechnol Biochem* 64(5):965–71.

Deuchi et al. 1995. Effect of the viscosity or deacetylation degree of chitosan on fecal fat excreted from rats fed on a high-fat diet. *Biosci Biotechnol Biochem* 59(5):781–85.

Kanauchi et al. 1995. Mechanism for the inhibition of fat digestion by chitosan and for the synergistic effect of ascorbate. *Biosci Biotechnol Biochem* 59(5):786–90.

Muzzarelli, R. 1999. Clinical and biochemical evaluation of chitosan for hypercholesterolemia and overweight control. *Chitin and Chitinases* 87:293–304.

Pittler et al. 1999. Randomized, double-blind trial of chitosan for body weight reduction. *Eur J Clin Nutr* 53(5):379–81.

Chondroitin sulfate

Definition: Chondroitin is a complex carbohydrate that is found in connective tissues in mammals. It attracts fluid to the joint and is necessary for joint flexibility and protection. Animal cartilage is the most significant known source of chondroitin, which is also present in human cartilage. Studies on chondroitin show that supplementation can not only ease joint pain and inflammation, but also repair damaged joint tissue.

Recommended for: osteoarthritis, torn ligaments and tendons, gout, headaches, lupus, HIV, bone healing and some viral infections

Scientific Updates: Japanese studies have found that the amount of chondroitin sulfate present in the synovial fluid found in the jaw joint can tell doctors the degree of damage and may help to determine the flexibility of such joints. It is also possible that chondroitin may boost bone healing and that it definitely seems to benefit people with forms of arthritic disease. Other studies suggest that it may also prevent the formation of blood clots, lower cholesterol and protect the cardiovascular system. Although we need more studies, we believe that coupling chondroitin with glucosamine sulfate is beneficial. There is also some evidence that the duo may be a potent inhibitor of the HIV virus.

Safety: Chondroitin is not recommended for children under the age of two. Nausea may result if taking more than 10 grams per day. It is safe to take glucosamine with chondroitin. There are no known drug interactions for chondroitin sulfate, but don't take chondroitin while using anticoagulant drugs. Also do not take chondroitin if you have a blood clotting disorder.

Product Forms: Stores sell chondroitin products most often in capsule form. Chondroitin is also frequently added to glucosamine in supplements designed to treat arthritis. Chondroitin may also be formulated with vitamin C. Most products range in potency from 400 to 600 mg.

Comments: Choose your chondroitin product wisely. Some products have been found to contain far less chondroitin than their labels claim. Children ages two to four may take chondroitin but should not take more than 10 grams per day. Typical dosage amounts range from 250 to 1,600 milligrams per day, but no official dosage guidelines currently exist. Chondroitin may work more effectively when coupled with glucosamine sulfate. For osteoarthritis, a typical dose is 400 mg three times per day.

References

Akama, H. and S. Saito. 2001. Glucosamine and chondroitin for osteoarthritis. *Arthritis Rheum* 45(1):107.

Bassleer et al. 1998. Effects of chondroitin sulfate and interleukin-1 beta on human articular chondrocytes cultivated in clusters. *Osteoarthritis Cartilage* 6(3):196–204.

Kerzberg et al. 1987. Combination of glycosaminoglycans and acetylsalicylic acid in knee osteoarthritis. *Scand J Rheum* 16:377.

Konlee, M. 1998. Sulfated polysaccharides (chondroitin sulfate and carrageenan) plus glucosamine sulfate are potent inhibitors of HIV. *Posit Health News* 17:4–7.

Moss et al. 1965. The effect of chondroitin sulfate on bone healing. *Oral Surg Oral Med Oral Pathol* 20:795–801.

Nishimura et al. 1998. Role of chondroitin sulfate-hyaluronan interactions in the viscoelastic properties of extracellular matrices and fluids. *Biochim Biophys Acta* 1380(1):1–9.

Okazaki et al. 1997. Chondroitin sulfate isomers in synovial fluid of healthy and diseased human temporomandibular joints. *Eur J Oral Sci* 105(5 Pt 1):440–43.

Coenzyme Q10 *(Co Q10, ubiquinone)*

Definition: Coenzyme Q10 (co Q10) is a substance that resembles vitamin E and is found in living cells. Like so many other emerging natural supplements, natural supplies of this particular compound decrease with age. Although coenzyme Q10 is found throughout the body, it is most highly concentrated in heart muscle cells. For this reason, replacing this compound may benefit heart-related conditions as well as other disorders by increasing nutrient, energy and oxygen supplies to heart muscle. It is also considered an antioxidant.

Recommended for: cardiovascular disease, congestive heart failure, mitral valve prolapse, cancer, gingivitis, high blood pressure, respiratory disease, asthma, mental illness, Alzheimer's disease, candida, obesity, multiple sclerosis, male infertility, periodontal disease, gastric ulcers, weakened immune systems and AIDS, chronic fatigue syndrome, breast cancer, leukemia

Scientific Updates: Recent studies have suggested that coenzyme Q10 supplementation may help to reduce high blood pressure, lower heart disease and boost immune defenses. Scientists are presently investigating coenzyme Q10 as a possible treatment for HIV; it may also be valuable for weight loss, gingivitis and even premature aging. It may benefit people suffering from certain kinds of cancer, especially leukemia and breast tumors. Its strongest application appears to be for heart-related problems, and one study reports that adding vitamin E to coenzyme Q10 was even more effective for artery disease.

Safety: A mild decrease in the effectiveness of warfarin (Coumadin), a blood thinning drug, has been reported with coenzyme Q10 supplementation. It may also decrease the effectiveness of some cholesterol-lowering drugs. Check with your doctor if you are on medications before taking this supplement. Congestive heart failure patients should consult their doctor before taking this supplement.

Product Forms: Capsules are the most common form of coenzyme Q10. Experts prefer solublized, oil-based products. Coenzyme Q10 is also commonly included in antioxidant combinations and cardiovascular formulations. Always look for pure, reliable sources of coenzyme Q10. Store supplements in a dark, cool environment.

Comments: Take coenzyme Q10 supplements with food. Taking it with a fat-containing food helps maximize its absorption. Common dosages range from 50 to 120 milligrams twice daily. There are some tests available that can check the level of coenzyme Q10 in your bloodstream.

References

Del Mar et al. 2001. Is coenzyme Q10 helpful for patients with idiopathic cardiomyopathy? *Med J Aust* 16:174(8):421.

Digiesi et al. 1992. Mechanism of action of coenzyme Q10 in essential hypertension. *Curr Ther Res* 51:668–72.

Kaikkonen et al. 1997. Effect of oral coenzyme Q10 on the oxidation resistance of human VLDL + LDL fraction: absorption and antioxidative properties of oil and granule-based preparations. *Free Radic Biol Med* 22:1195–1202.

Lockwood et al. 1995. Progress on therapy of breast cancer with vitamin Q10 and the regression of metastases. *Biochem Biophys Res Comm* 212:172–77.

Morisco et al. 1993. Effect of coenzyme Q10 in patients with congestive heart failure: a long-term multicenter randomized study. *Clin Invest* 71:S134–36.

Thomas et al. 2001. Dietary cosupplementation with vitamin E and coenzyme Q(10) inhibits atherosclerosis in apolipoprotein E gene knockout mice. *Arterioscler Thromb Vasc Biol* 21(4):585–93.

Creatine

Definition: Creatine is considered a naturally occurring nutrient found in skeletal muscles. Three amino acids (arginine, glycine and methionine) comprise creatine. Creatine assists in providing muscle fibers with the energy needed to facilitate quick and forceful movements. The body obtains most of its creatine through dietary sources; however, some people now use a supplement form of creatine to enhance muscle building and athletic performance. Several clinical studies suggest that creatine supplementation allows for more energy storage, increased stamina and strength, as well as synthesis of protein and lean muscle mass.

Recommended for: athletic endurance, muscle building, weight loss

Scientific Updates: Studies have shown that taking creatine orally does enhance muscle performance during intense resistance exercise with an increase of body mass. One study concluded that creatine supplementation helped to enhance exercise output and created better performance in repetitive bench presses. There is also some evidence that creatine lowers cholesterol and may protect against bone loss.

Safety: No significant long-term studies on the safety of creatine exist. Using it for an increase in muscle mass is considered relatively safe. Short-term side effects reported by athletes using large doses of creatine include diarrhea, gas, muscle cramping and intestinal upset. Anyone suffering from any medical problem should not use creatine without a physician's approval. People suffering from kidney disorders should not take creatine. It may also cause dehydration.

Product Forms: The way to best use creatine is in powder form. You can obtain exact measurements with specific dispensing cups contained in powdered forms. Companies often add it to energy and muscle building formulas.

Comments: Athletes typically take creatine in 5-gram doses taken four times daily for a week, then reduced to 2 to 5 grams daily. This can be rather costly, and many coaches and experts don't sanction the use of creatine for their athletes until more scientific evidence emerges.

References

Benzi, G. and A. Ceci. 2001. Creatine as nutritional supplementation and medicinal product. *J Sports Med Phys Fitness* 41(1):1–10.

Burke et al. 2000. The effect of continuous low dose creatine supplementation on force, power, and total work. *Int J Sport Nutr Exerc Metab* 10(3):235–44.

Persky, A. and G. Brazeau. 2001. Clinical pharmacology of the dietary supplement creatine monohydrate. *Pharmacol Rev* 53(2):161–76.

Rockwell et al. 2001. Creatine supplementation affects muscle creatine during energy restriction. *Med Sci Sports Exerc* 33(1):61–8.

Volek et al. 1997. Creatine supplementation enhances muscular performance during high intensity resistance exercise. *Journal of American Dietetic Association* 97:765–770.

DHA *(Docosahexaenoic Acid)*

Definition: Docosahexaenoic acid (DHA) is a member of the omega-3 essential fatty acids and is found in cold-water fish like salmon, mackerel, herring, sardines and albacore tuna. It is thought that the modern diet is lacking in all the omega-3 fatty acids, which may explain, in part, the higher incidence of cardiovascular disease in the United States. DHA can decrease blood fats and may also help with various neurological disorders.

Recommended for: atherosclerosis, heart disease, high cholesterol, ADHD, mental disorders, depression, inflammatory conditions.

Scientific Updates: DHA in breast milk is a vital nutrient for a healthy nervous system and for normal vision in babies. DHA supplementation for premature infants demonstrated significant benefits for brain functions. New studies also suggest that DHA supplementation may help with hyperactivity or aggressive behavior and for depression. It also appears to have natural anti-inflammatory properties, making it desirable for joint diseases, etc. Low DHA levels have been linked to Alzheimer's disease.

Safety: With large doses of fish oil or DHA, some elevation in blood sugar has been reported. It has, in rare instances, raised LDL levels in some people. Pregnant women or those trying to conceive should not use cod liver oil as a source of DHA. DHA alone does not have the blood thinning effect of EPA, another fatty acid found in cold-water fish.

Product Forms: Stores sell DHA most commonly in capsules, often as part of an essential fatty acid array.

Comments: Most scientific data was obtained using doses ranging from 1 to 3 grams of DHA daily from a fish oil source. Vitamin E is often included in fish oil supplements to prevent oxidation, although this effect is in question. Microalgae sources of vegetarian DHA are also available. Most fish oil supplements contain between 10 and 12 percent DHA. DHA is commonly paired with EPA, another essential fatty acid found in cold-water fish. Using pectin with fish oil supplementation may help to lower cholesterol levels more effectively.

References

Davidson et al. 1997. Effects of docosahexaenoic acid on serum lipoproteins in patients with combined hyperlipidemia: A randomized, double-blind, placebo-controlled trial. *J Am Coll Nutr* 16(3):236–43.

Gibson, R.A., M.A. Neumann, and M. Makrides. 1996. Effect of dietary docosahexaenoic acid on brain composition and neural function in term infants. *Lipids* 31:177S–81S.

Hamazaki et al. 1996. The effect of docosahexaenoic acid on aggression in young adults. A placebo-controlled double-blind study. *J Clin Invest* 97:1129–33.

Jorgensen et al. 2001. Is there a relation between docosahexaenoic acid concentration in mothers' milk and visual development in term infants. *J Pediatr Gastroenterol Nutr* 32(3):293–6.

Nelson et al. 1997. The effect of dietary docosahexaenoic acid on platelet function, platelet fatty acid composition, and blood coagulation in humans. *Lipids* 32:1129–36.

Soderberg et al. 1991. Fatty acid composition of brain phospholipids in aging and in Alzheimer's disease. *Lipids* 26:421–25.

Stevens et al. 1995. Essential fatty acid metabolism in boys with attention-deficit hyperactivity disorder. *Am J Clin Nutr* 62:761–68.

DHEA *(Dehydroepiandrosterone)*

Definition: DHEA is the most abundant hormone found in mammals. Scientists use it to make all steroidal hormones, including estrogens, androgens and corticosteroids. Our adrenal glands produce DHEA from a hormone called pregnenolone. DHEA production is highest at age twenty-five and then continuously declines to approximately 20 percent of peak age by seventy-five. Although numerous studies (animal) suggest that it may benefit people with cancer, diabetes, immune dysfunction, etc., no long-term human studies have confirmed these effects. 7-KETO DHEA (a metabolite of DHEA) may have equal potential with less risk of side effects.

Recommended for: lupus, rheumatoid arthritis, depression, psoriasis, diabetes, prostate disease, menopause, high cholesterol, obesity, geriatric conditions

Scientific Updates: More than one study suggests that DHEA improved the physical and emotional status of older test subjects with no apparent side effects. Other studies have shown that it also appears to increase muscle strength and lean body mass and that it boosts immune function. DHEA may also prevent or treat lupus and may protect against osteoporosis. Preliminary data of 7-KETO DHEA show that it may increase the burning of fat and may enhance memory.

Safety: DHEA supplementation should be done with the consent of your physician. While no significant reactions have occurred to supplementation, some minor acne has occurred in some people. I don't recommend DHEA for anyone suffering from breast, ovarian, uterine or prostate cancer, since these can be hormonally stimulated malignancies. It is also not for pregnant or nursing women or for children or adolescents. Experts caution against extended use of large amounts of DHEA (over 50 mg/day). Women taking over 25 mg daily may experience excessive hair growth. DHEA may also stimulate the growth of undetected breast or prostate tumors. It is not for people with liver disease or breast or prostate cancer or a history of these diseases. The safety of 7-KETO DHEA currently under testing.

Product Forms: DHEA and 7-KETO DHEA (a metabolite of DHEA) are available in capsules and tablets. DHEA is sometimes synthesized from Mexican wild yam through a laboratory process.

Comments: Taking Mexican wild yam alone will not supply the body with DHEA. Replacing isolated hormones into the body through supplementation offers a great deal of promise; however, scientists have not yet assessed its long-term effects in humans.

References

Barrett-Connor et al. 1990. Dehydroepiandrosterone sulfate and breast cancer risk. *Cancer Research* 50(20):6571-4.

Barrett-Connor et al. 1993. A prospective study of dehydroepiandrosterone sulfate (DHEAS) and bone mineral density in older men and women. *Am J Epidemiology* 137(2):201-6.

Callies et al. 2001. Dehydroepiandrosterone replacement in women with adrenal insufficiency: effects on body composition, serum leptin, bone turnover, and exercise capacity. *J Clin Endocrinal Metab* 86(5):1968-72.

Kuebler et al. 2001. Dehydroepiandrosterone restores hepatocellular function and prevents liver damage in estrogen-deficient females following trauma and hemorrhage. *J Surg Research* 97(2):196-201.

Morales et al. 1994. Effects of replacement dose of dehydroepiandrosterone in men and women of advancing age. *J Clin Endocrinol Metab* 78(6):1360-7.

Wolkowitz et al. 1995. Antidepressant and cognition-enhancing effects of DHEA in major depression. *Ann NY Acad Sci* 774:337-9.

DMAE (Dimethylaminoethanol)

Defintion: DMAE is a compound that occurs naturally in the body and can be found in some foods. It is often paired with choline or phosphatidylchlorine for its effect as a brain tonic and as a mild stimulant on the nervous system. Its most popular current use is for mood elevation, increased mental performance and enhanced energy. It may also increase longevity and may hold value for Alzheimer's disease, although those effects are still considered unproven. It does have a history of use for ADHD and other behavioral disorders.

Recommended for: learning disorders, ADHD, depression, Alzheimer's disease, senile dementia, memory disorders

Scientific Updates: There is some evidence that DMAE does improve concentration and memory skills. Scientists believe that it converts to choline in the brain, which boosts the production of acetylcholine, thereby enhancing cognitive function, memory and mood. It also serves as an antioxidant in brain cells and protects them against certain harmful toxins. One study confirms it also creates more vivid or lucid dreams.

Safety: Headaches, leg cramps and muscle spasms have been reported with DMAE use. Large doses can cause anxiety, nervousness, insomnia and increased blood pressure. Women who are pregnant or breastfeeding, those with convulsions, epilepsy and manic-depressive illness should not use DMAE.

Product Forms: DMAE comes in 100 mg capsules and in liquid supplements. It may also be found in formulas for brain enhancement, depression or ADHD.

Comments: Like DHEA, the long-term use of DMAE in humans has not yet been properly assessed. Although, some studies are promising, there is still much research that needs to be conducted.

References

Dimpfel et al. 1996. Source density analysis of functional topographical EEG: monitoring of cognitive drug action. *Eur J Med Res* 1(6):283–90.

Hochschild, R. 1973. Effect of demethylaminoethyl p-chlorophenoxyacetate on the life span of male Swiss Webster albino mice. *Experimental Gerontology* 8:177–83.

Nikolova-Karakashian et al. 1997. Sphingomyelin metabolism in rat liver after chronic dietary replacement of choline by N-aminodeanol. *J Lipid Res* 38(9):1764–70.

Sergio et al. 1988. Use of DMAE (2-dimethylaminoethanol) in the induction of lucid dreams. *Med Hypotheses* 26(4):255–7.

Essential Fatty Acids

Definition: Also known as vitamin F, these fatty acids (omega-6 and omega-3) must be supplied through the diet. The body cannot produce them alone. Cold-water fish contain two essential fatty acids referred to as EPA and DHA. Flaxseed and fish oil are rich in omega-3 factors. GLA (gamma-linoleic acid) is found in evening primrose oil. Omega-6 fatty acids are found in several vegetable oils (black currant seed, borage, flaxseed, soy, walnut and evening primrose oil).

Recommended for: high blood pressure, heart disease, arthritis, breast cancer, psoriasis, eczema, weight loss, multiple sclerosis, brain function, PMS, inflammatory conditions, ADHD, prostate protection, depression

Scientific Updates: Both classes of the omega fatty acids have been shown to significantly reduce the risk of cardiovascular disease, contribute to nerve health and act as natural anti-inflammatory agents. New studies confirm their prostate protective action and their beneficial effect in breast tissue (especially the omega-3 class). Scientist now believe a deficiency in fatty acids may cause depression and ADHD.

Safety: Diabetics should not take fish oil, but experts recommend other sources of essential fatty acids including fresh cold-water fish. Anyone with hormonally related cancers should limit their intake of primrose oil and use black currant oil instead.

Product Forms: Essential fatty acids come in loose liquids or capsulized liquid forms and often offer a variety of types from DHA, EPA and CLA. They are also available in flaxseed and evening primrose oil supplements.

Comments: You are much more likely to consume an excess of omega-6 fats that omega-3. A balance between the two is optimal. Add flaxseed oil to other foods. The oil is especially good for children, who may be deficient in fatty acids.

References

Collett et al. 2001. N-6 and N-3 polyunsaturated fatty acids differentially modulate oncogenic Ras activation in colonocytes. *Am J Physiol Cell Physiol* 280(5):C1066–75.

Hughes-Fulford et al. 2001. Fatty acid regulates gene expression and growth of human prostate cancer PC-3 cells. *Carcinogenesis* 22(5):701–7.

Vermunt et al. 2001. Dietary trans alpha-linolenic acid from deodorised rapeseed oil and plasma lipids and lipoproteins in healthy men: the TransLinE Study. *Br J Nutr* 85(3):387–92.

Evening Primrose Oil

Definition: Evening primrose oil (EPO) is a rich source of GLA (Gamma-linoleic acid) which is a powerful natural anti-inflammatory compound made from omega-6 fatty acids. In turn, the body uses GLA to make an anti-inflammatory messenger chemical (PGE-1). GLA is found in the omega-6 fatty acids (safflower oil and others).

Recommended for: fibrocystic breast disease, rheumatoid arthritis, diabetic neuropathy, cardiovascular disease, eczema, lupus, psoriasis, MS, menstrual disorders, menopause

Scientific Updates: Although there is still some question as to whether EPO really benefits, eczema, PMS, hyperactivity and MS, it has shown the ability to inhibit blood clotting, lower cholesterol and reduce inflammation, especially in arthritic conditions. It may also be of benefit to people with menstrual disorders like schizophrenia and may inhibit the abnormal cell division seen in cancer.

Safety: Supplemental EPO is generally regarded as safe but should not be taken by people on blood thinning drugs without their doctor's consent. A safe diet should also incorporate the omega-3 fatty acids from fish oil, olive oil, etc.

Product Forms: EPO is available in capsules and in concentrated oil products. It is often added to women's products and can also be found in creams and lotions.

Comments: Be aware that the action of EPO can be blocked by high consumption of saturated fats or by a lack of vitamin C, magnesium, zinc and the B-vitamins. I recommend taking EPO as a part of a supplement with a variety of essential fatty acids.

References

Belch, J. and A. Hill. 2000. Evening primrose oil and borage oil in rheumatologic conditions. *Am J Clin Nutr* 71(1 Suppl):352S–352S.

Charnock, J. 2000. Gamma-linoleic acid provides additional protection against ventricular fibrillation in aged rats fed linoleic acid rich diets. *Prostaglandins Leukot Fatty Acids* 62(2):1239–34.

Head et al. 2000. Prevention of nerve conduction deficit in diabetic rats by polyunsaturated fatty acids. *Am J Clin Nutr* 71(1 Suppl):386S–392S.

Horrobin, D. 2000. Essential fatty acid metabolism and its modification in atopic eczema. *Am J Clin Nutr* 71(1 Suppl):367S–72S.

Joy et al. 2000. Polyunsaturated fatty acid (fish or evening primrose oil) for schizophrenia. *Cochrane Database Syst Rev* (2):CD001257.

Fiber

Definition: Fiber refers to the indigestible portions of all plants, many of which we eat. It is not found in animal foods. Two types of fiber, soluble and insoluble, are important for human health. Soluble fiber dissolves in water and acts like a gel in the colon to soften the stool and promote a feeling of fullness. Insoluble fiber does not dissolve and has strong laxative actions due to its ability to hold water and move waste through the bowel.

Recommended for: cardiovascular health, high cholesterol, cancer prevention, varicose veins, hemorrhoids, constipation, colon cancer, breast cancer, diverticulosis, diabetes, obesity, Parkinson's disease, irritable bowel syndrome, indigestion, high blood pressure

Scientific Updates: Soluble fiber can lower cholesterol and may also decrease the amount of insulin needed to deal with blood sugar levels. Soluble fiber promotes feelings of fullness and can help with weight loss. High-fiber diets may decrease the risk of colon and breast cancer, ease constipation and irritable bowel syndrome, and help prevent diverticulosis, hemorrhoids, high cholesterol and diabetes. It is particularly important for children, whose diets are often low in fiber.

Safety: Fiber is considered safe if it is in dietary form and not taken in such excess that diarrhea or obstruction could occur. Drink plenty of water when taking fiber, and if you suffer from any type of colon disorder or digestive system disease, check with your doctor before adding a fiber supplement. If you don't drink enough water, you raise your chances of bloating and constipation. Take vitamins and mineral supplements at different times than fiber because nutrient absorption may be impaired. Do not use fiber if you have trouble swallowing. Psyllium products can cause gas.

Product Forms: Fiber comes in tablets, powders, bars, etc. Bran fiber has low solubility with good water-holding properties. Psyllium has an insoluble seed around which forms colorless transparent mucilage. Gums form a homogenous adhesive gelatinous mass to expedite waste transit. Methyl cellulose has slow solubility and creates a viscous solution for expulsion. Isphagula husk swells rapidly to form a mucilage. In general, soluble fibers are found in fruits, oats, barley and legumes (beans). Psyllium, gums, mucilages, glucomannan and pectins are soluble fibers. Insoluble fibers are found in vegetables, grains like wheat, brans and flaxseed.

Comments: Few of us eat the recommended 25 to 45 grams of fiber per day, so supplementation is a good idea. Drink at least 8 ounces of water for each tablespoon of fiber that you take.

References

Alabaster et al. 1997. Inhibition by wheat bran cereals of the development of aberrant crypt foci and colon tumours. *Food Chem Toxicol* 35(5):517–22.

Fruhbeck, G. 1996. Dietary fiber and coronary heart disease prevention. JAMA. 26:275(24):1883.

Jenkins et al. 2001. Effect of a very high-fiber vegetable, fruit, and nut diet on serum lipids and colonic function. *Metabolism* 50(4):494–503.

Slavin, J. 1994. Epidemiological evidence for the impact of whole grains on health. *Crit Rev Food Sci Nutr* 34(5–6):427–34.

Sutton et al. 2000. Recommending high-fiber diets to prevent colorectal cancer. *Med Health R I* 83(8):259–60.

Williams, C. 1995. Importance of dietary fiber in childhood. J Am Diet Assoc. 95(10):1140–6.

Glucosamine

Definition: Glucosamine sulfate holds some very exciting potential as a safe treatment for osteoarthritis and other inflammatory joint conditions. It is a naturally occurring amino monosaccharide found in the joints of mammals. Glucosamine enables the body to manufacture a mucopolysaccharide called glycosaminoglycan found in cartilage. When taken as a dietary supplement, glucosamine appears to be able to significantly support the rebuilding of damaged cartilage.

Recommended for: arthritis (especially osteoarthritis), cartilage injury, connective tissue disease, joint pain, TMJ

Scientific Updates: A glucosamine deficiency has been linked to osteoarthritis. Some studies support the ability of glucosamine to act as a healing, anti-inflammatory, disease-modifying agent. This makes it superior to NSAIDs. Although long-term studies have yet to be done, some twenty clinical trials have showed that glucosamine sulfate can gradually reduce pain while improving range of motion and walking speed in people with osteoarthritis. In addition to possibly alleviating symptoms of osteoarthritis, glucosamine sulfate may also benefit wounds and kidney stones. Studies have found that 1,500 mg per day of glucosamine for four weeks was more effective and much better tolerated than the conventional drug, ibuprofen. Glucosamine may reverse the progression of degenerative joint disease and appears to have powerful antiviral properties against HIV when combined with chondroitin.

Safety: At doses of 1,500 mg daily, no toxicity has been reported. Be aware that some glucosamine supplements contain sodium chloride (salt), which is contraindicated in people with high blood pressure or other diseases. Some people have experienced short-term gastrointestinal upset, sleepiness, headaches or rashes after taking glucosamine.

Product Forms: Glucosamine comes in capsules and tablets commonly sold in 250 to 750 mg potencies. Liquid products are also available. Frequently, glucosamine is combined with chondroitin for maximum effect. Look for the sulfate form of glucosamine.

Comments: An average dose of glucosamine for anyone with osteoarthritis is 500 mg three times daily.

References

Brief et al. 2001. Use of glucosamine and chondroitin sulfate in the management of osteoarthritis. *J Am Acad Orthop Surg* 9(2):71–8.

Da Camara, C. and G. Dowless. 1998. Glucosamine sulfate for osteoarthritis. *Ann Pharmacother* 32(5):580–87.

Kelly, G. 1998. The role of glucosamine sulfate and chondroitin sulfates in the treatment of degenerative joint disease. *Altern Med Rev* 3(1):27–39.

Konlee, M. 1998. Sulfated polysaccharides (chondroitin sulfate and carrageenan) plus glucosamine sulfate are potent inhibitors of HIV. *Posit Health News* 17:4–7.

Qiu et al. 1998. Efficacy and safety of glucosamine sulfate versus ibuprofen in patients with knee osteoarthritis *Arzneimittelforschung* 48(5):469–74.

Towheed et al. 2001. Glucosamine therapy for treating osteoarthritis (Cochrane Review). *Cochrane Database Syst Rev* 1:CD002946.

Hydroxycitric Acid (HCA)

Definition: Found in the garcinia cambogia fruit, HCA is a form of citric acid that inhibits the ability of the liver to make fats from carbohydrates. When HCA is present, carbohydrates convert to glycogen stores rather than fat stores. This contributes to better energy reserves, more stamina and increased weight control.

Recommended for: obesity, appetite control, weight loss and maintenance and possibly diabetes

Scientific Updates: Preliminary research studies suggest that HCA may be useful for weight loss. Laboratory trials have found that it can decrease the conversion of carbohydrates into fat stores by inhibiting the action of specific enzymes. It also appears to suppress the appetite. One study reported that consuming 1 gram of the fruit prior to each meal resulted in a weight loss of 1 pound per day. Other studies have questioned this effect.

Safety: HCA has not been linked to any adverse side effects or drug interactions at this writing.

Product Forms: HCA supplements are available in tablets, capsules, powders, snack bars, chewing gum and weight-loss meal replacements. HCA is commonly added to other compounds in weight-loss formulas.

Comments: Be aware that the amounts of HCA used in studies were much greater than the typical 1,500 mg taken daily.

References

Greenwood et al. 1981. Effect of (-)-hydroxycitrate on development of obesity in the Zucker obese rat. *Am Phys J* 240:E72–78.

Heymsfield et al. 1998. Garcinia cambogia (hydroxycitric acid) as a potential antiobesity agent. *JAMA* 280:1596–1600.

Lowenstein, J. 1971. Effect of (-)-hydroxycitrate on fatty acid synthesis by rat liver in vivo. *J Biol Chem* 246(3):629–32.

Mattes, R. and L. Bormann. 2000. Effects of (-)-hydroxycitric acid on appetitive variables. *Physiol Behav* 71(1–2):87–94.

Seroy, S. 1999. Response to JAMA HCA report. *Townsend Letter for Doctors and Patients* Feb/Mar:120–21

Triscari, J. and A. Sullivan. 1977. Comparative effects of (-)-hydroxycitrate and (=)-allo-hydroxycitrate on acetyl CoA carboxylase and fatty acid and cholesterol synthesis in vivo. *Lipids* 12(4):357–63.

Lecithin

Definition: Lecithin is a vital compound necessary to maintain the health of cell membranes. Membranes are crucial because they largely regulate life-preserving processes on a cellular level. Lecithin is comprised of choline, a B-vitamin, and also contains inositol and linoleic acid. Although it is technically a fatty substance, lecithin works to emulsify fats and is important in preventing arteriosclerosis and cardiovascular disease. It also contributes to better brain function. Lecithin expedites the removal of fats from the body. Most lecithin is commercially extracted from soybeans or egg sources.

Recommended for: AIDS, herpes, chronic fatigue, MS, arteriosclerosis, high cholesterol, heart disease, high blood pressure, obesity, Alzheimer's disease

Scientific Updates: Lecithin is sometimes considered a memory enhancer because it contains choline. Choline enhances cognitive functions and may help improve short term memory and prevent memory loss. Research has shown a link between acetylcholine deficiency and Alzheimer's disease. Although we need more studies, we know it may help diseases like MS, which have been related to abnormal fat metabolism.

Safety: Large doses of lecithin may cause diarrhea and nausea. Follow product label instructions, and do not exceed recommended dosages.

Product Forms: Stores sell lecithin in granule form or as a capsulized substance either alone or in combination with other nutrients like glucomannan.

Comments: Lecithin is commonly added to fatty acid supplements or products designed to support the central nervous system.

References

Thal et al. 1983. Oral physostigmine and lecithin improve memory in Alzheimer disease. *Ann Neurol* 13(5):491–6.

Wecker, L. 1986. Neurochemical effects of choline supplementation. *Can J Physiol Pharmacol* 64(3):329–33.

Lutein

Definition: Lutein is an antioxidant that belongs to the carotenoid family and is found in leafy green vegetables. It is also present in the macula or center section of the retina of the eye where it serves to protect the retina from ultra-violet light damage. Today, science considers it a valuable nutrient for any macular disorder and to protect against macular degeneration, a major cause of blindness in older individuals.

Recommended for: secondary macular degeneration, cataracts, night blindness, retinal injury, glaucoma, visual disturbances

Scientific Updates: One study reported that people with the highest dietary intake of lutein had a 57 percent decreased risk of developing macular degeneration compared with those who had the lowest consumption of lutein. The same type of correlation was also seen with cataracts. Lutein may also protect the colon and prostate from cancer.

Safety: No toxicity or drug interactions have been found at this writing.

Product Forms: Lutein is available as a single supplement or as part of vision enhancing or antioxidant formulas.

Comments: Approximately 6 mg of lutein per day is thought to afford retinal protection. If you take lutein in supplemental form, take it with meals for optimal absorption.

References

Giovannucci et al. 1995. Intake of carotenoids and retinol in relation to risk of prostate cancer. *J Natl Cancer Inst* 6:87(23):1767–76.

Hammond et al. 2001. Carotenoids in the retina and lens: possible acute and chronic effects on human visual performance. *Arch Biochem Biophys* 1:385(1):41–6.

Hankinson et al. 1992. Nutrient intake and cataract extraction in women: A prospective study. *Br Med J* 305:335–39.

Landrum, J. and R. Bone. 2001. Lutein, zeaxanthin, and the macular pigment. *Arch Biochem Biophys* J 1:385(1):28–40.

Natural therapies for ocular disorders, part two: cataracts and glaucoma. 2001. *Altern Med Rev* 6(2):141–66.

Seddon et al. 1994. Dietary carotenoids, vitamins A, C, and E, and advanced age-related macular degeneration. *JAMA* 272:1413–20.

Slattery et al. 2000. Carotenoids and colon cancer. *Am J Clin Nutr* 71(2):575–582.

Lycopene

Definition: Lycopene is a nutrient found primarily in tomatoes and like lutein, is a member of the carotenoid family, which gives it powerful antioxidant actions. Watermelon and guava also contain lycopene. Lycopene is considered the most cancer-protective compound belonging to the carotenoid family.

Recommended for: cancer protection (especially the prostate, lung, gastrointestinal tract, cervix and colon), eye health and protection, radiation exposure, prostate health, smokers

Scientific Updates: Lycopene has clearly been associated with prostate cancer protection, especially at levels of 6.5 mg per daily. This amount demonstrated a 21 percent decreased risk of prostate cancer compared with those eating the least amount of lycopene. Eating tomato-based foods resulted in similar findings. Although there is no scientific data that lycopene benefits benign prostatic hyperplasia (BPH), it only stands to reason that it could due to the fact that lycopene is the most abundant carotenoid found in the prostate gland. Another study found that low tomato intake was also linked to higher risk for gastrointestinal tract cancer. In addition, women who did not eat tomatoes had almost 5 times greater risk of cervical cancer. The same type of correlation applies to breast cancer and heart disease as well. Lycopene also boosts immune function by increasing killer-T cells. Tomatoes also appear to protect the eyes from light damage and the body from radiation exposure.

Safety: No adverse effects or toxicity have been reported with lycopene, and there are no known drug interactions at this writing.

Product Forms: Lycopene is available as a single supplement but is commonly added to multiple vitamin, mineral and antioxidant formulas.

Comments: If you dislike tomatoes, you are likely to be low on lycopene and should take supplementation. Recommended dosages of this nutrient have not been established; however, in some studies, 6.5 mg per day were required to achieve optimal protective effects. It is unclear whether tomato juice has the same protective effects as the whole tomato or concentrated tomato products.

References

Corridan et al. 1998. Carotenoids and immune response in elderly people. *Proc Nutr Soc* 57:3A.

Djuric, Z. and L. Powell. 2001. Antioxidant capacity of lycopene-containing foods. *Int J Food Sci Nutr* 52(2):143–9.

Dorgan et al. 1998. Relationships of serum carotenoids, retinol, alpha-tocopherol, and selenium with breast cancer risk: results from a prospective study in Columbia, Missouri. *Cancer Causes Control* 9:89–97.

Franceshci et al. 1994. Tomatoes and risk of digestive-tract cancers. *Int J Cancer* 59:181–84.

Giovannucci et al. 1995. Intake of carotenoids and retinol in relation to risk of prostate cancer. *J Natl Cancer Inst* 87:1767–76.

Kim et al. 2000. Chemoprevention of lung cancer by lycopene. *Biofactors* 13(1–4):95–102.

Kohlmeyer et al. 1997. Lycopene and myocardial infarction risk in the EUROMIC study. *Am J Epidemiol* 146:618–26.

Levy et al. 1995. Lycopene is a more potent inhibitory of human cancer cell proliferation than either beta-carotene or beta-carotene. *Nutr Cancer* 24:257–66.

Saada, Helen and Khaled Azab. 2001. S Role of lycopene in recovery of radiation induced injury to mammalian cellular organelles. *Pharmazie* 56(3):239–41.

Stahl et al. 2001. Dietary tomato paste protects against ultraviolet light-induced erythema in humans. *J Nutr* 131(5):1449–51.

de la Taille et al. 2001. Cancer of the prostate: influence of nutritional factors. Vitamins, antioxidants and trace elements. *Presse Med* 24:30(11):557–60.

Van Eenwyk et al. 1991. Dietary and serum carotenoids and cervical intraepithelial neoplasia. *Int J Cancer* 48:34–38.

Malic Acid

Definition: Malic acid is a compound involved in the conversion of carbohydrates to energy. Although the body naturally produces malic acid, it is also found in various fruits and vegetables. Apples are rich in malic acid, which may explain the old proverb that "an apple a day keeps the doctor away." Today, malic acid supplements have value for muscle disorders.

Recommended for: fibromyalgia, muscle strains, backaches, muscle metabolism diseases, recovery after strenuous activity

Scientific Updates: Some preliminary data suggests that people with fibromyalgia might have difficulty producing or using malic acid which could interfere with normal muscle function. Although some studies suggest the value of malic acid in supplement form, others question its value. More trials are needed to establish its value for fibromyalgia, although anecdotal evidence backs its use. One study did establish that malic acid combined with magnesium taken over six months at a dose of 1,600 mg of malic acid and 400 mg of magnesium did result in significant improvement. There is also some evidence that malic acid may help muscles to recover faster after strenuous physical activity.

Safety: Malic acid seems safe at recommended dosages. Lose stools at higher doses have been reported. Its safety for pregnant or nursing women, children, or people with severe liver or kidney disease has not been established.

Product Availability: Although malic acid is available as a single supplement, it is most often used in combinations designed to treat muscle disorders like fibromyalgia. Make sure that your are getting enough of the malic acid daily (as based on studies) to accomplish results.

Comments: The usual therapeutic dose of malic acid for fibromyalgia is 1,200 to 2,800 mg per day which is often combined with 400 mg magnesium and other compounds.

References

Abraham, G. and J. Flechas. 1992. Management of fibromyalgia: rationale for the use of magnesium and malic acid. *J Nutr Med* 3:49–59.

Dunaev et al. 1988. Effect of malic acid salts on physical work capacity and its recovery after exhausting muscular activity. *Farmakol Toksikol* 51(3):21–5.

Fiume, Z. 2001. Final report on the safety assessment of Malic Acid and Sodium Malate. *Int J Toxicol* 20 Suppl 1:47–55.

Russell et al. 1995. Treatment of fibromyalgia syndrome with Super Malic®: a randomized, double blind, placebo controlled, crossover pilot study. *J Rheumatol* 22:953–958.

MSM *(methylsulfonyl methane)*

Definition: MSM is a naturally occurring compound that is considered a source of dietary sulfur, needed to produce muscles, skin, hair and nails. MSM is usually derived from another compound called dimethyl sulfoxide (DMSO). MSM plays a variety of roles in the body and has caught the attention of scientists for its ability to detoxify cells, which helps to inhibit allergic reactions to pollen and to decrease pain and inflammation seen in arthritis, tendinitis, muscle sprains. MSM levels in the body decline with age.

Recommended for: sore muscles, fibromyalgia, allergies, detoxification, chronic fatigue, psoriasis, acne, constipation, heartburn, lupus, breast cancer, arthritis, gout

Scientific Updates: Some studies have found that oral doses of DMSO and MSM reduce the destruction caused by arthritis in animal test subjects. Other studies suggest that it may protect against autoimmune diseases. It has also been recognized as playing a key role in people receiving bone marrow transplants. Sulfur also plays a major role in the function of insulin and may help to decrease pollen allergies by blocking the allergens from entering the cell membrane. It also has powerful antioxidant effects, fights giardia and boosts immune responses.

Safety: There is no apparent toxicity in MSM. Some people have experienced mild diarrhea, headache, and fatigue, which may result from initial cell detoxification. MSM does not cause the sulfur breath associated with DMSO.

Product Forms: MSM is available in 500 to 1,000 mg capsules and tablets, and also comes in powdered supplements. It is often combined with chondroitin, glucosamine sulfate, vitamin C, magnesium for joint and muscle disorders.

Comments: MSM experts suggest starting at 2 to 4 grams (2,000 to 4,000 mg) daily for several days and working up to 8 grams per day until symptoms improve. Lower your dosage if stomach upset occurs.

References

Egorin et al. 1998. Plasma concentrations and pharmacokinetics of dimethylsulfoxide and its metabolites in patients undergoing peripheral-blood stem-cell transplants. *J Clin Oncol* 16(2):610–15.

Morton, J. and B. Siegel. 1986. Effects of oral dimethyl sulfoxide and dimethyl sulfone on murine autoimmune lymphoproliferative disease. *Proc Soc Exp Biol Med* 183(2):227–30.

Muravev et al. 1991. Effect of dimethyl sulfoxide and dimethyl sulfone on a destructive process in the joints of mice with spontaneous arthritis. *Patol Fiziol Eksp Ter* 2:37–39.

Melatonin

Definition: Melatonin is a naturally occurring hormone secreted by the pineal gland in the mid-brain. Darkness triggers the production of melatonin, which in turn brings on sleep. Experts believe melatonin regulates the body's internal clock. The experts also link it to anti-aging properties; melatonin also may inhibit the growth of some types of cancer, may slow the progression of the HIV virus, and may play an integral role in cardiovascular health. Its full chemical name is N-acetyl-5-methoxy-tryptamine.

Recommended for: aging-related disorders, insomnia, jet lag, weak immune system, high cholesterol, arteriosclerosis, mental illness, cancer prevention, osteoporosis prevention, lung cancer

Scientific Updates: Melatonin is best known for its ability to promote sleep especially when changing time zones. It is also thought to have beneficial effects on aging and immune function. Other studies suggest that it may slow metastatic lung cancer and protect cells from free radical damage while boosting the activity of glutathione peroxidase, a very important protectant compound. It is also thought to contribute to the release of growth and sex hormones and may prevent osteoporosis.

Safety: Several studies have established the relative safety of taking melatonin supplements, although scientists still have to assess long-term effects. At this writing, it has no known toxicity even in relatively high amounts. Some individuals have experienced strange dreams or a feeling of short-term depression or grogginess following a nighttime dose. I don't recommend melatonin for pregnant or nursing mothers or for anyone suffering from severe allergies, leukemia, lymphoma, autoimmune diseases or severe depression. Anyone who is taking antidepressants or who is trying to conceive should not take melatonin. Use caution when giving the supplement to children. Do not mix melatonin with alcohol, sedative drugs or antidepressants without your doctor's approval.

Product Forms: Melatonin is usually sold in capsulized form and is often added in sleep formulas that contain other sedative herbs.

Comments: Research indicates that 0.5 to 5 mg, taken one to two hours before bedtime, works well for most cases of insomnia or jet lag. Melatonin is available in lower doses now so you start with a small dose and work up.

References

Bonilla et al. 2001. Melatonin prolongs survival of immunodepressed mice infected with the Venezuelan equine encephalomyelitis virus. *Trans R Soc Trop Med Hyg* 95(2):207–10.

Hardeland et al. 1993. The significance of the metabolism of the neurohormone melatonin: antioxidative protection and formation of bioactive substances. *Neuroscience and Biobehavioral Reviews* 17:347–357.

Hill, S. and D. Glask. 1998. Effect of the pineal hormone melatonin on the proliferation and morphological characteristics of human breast cancer cells. (MCF7) in culture. *Cancer Research* 48:6121–6126.

Katz, G. 2001. Exogenous melatonin, jet lag, and psychosis: preliminary case results. *J Clin Psychopharmacol* 21(3):349–51.

Lesnikov et al. 1994. Pineal cross-transplantation as evidence for an endogenous aging clock. *Annals NY Academy of Sciences* 719:456–460.

MacFarlane et al. 1991. The effects of exogenous melatonin on the total sleep time and daytime alertness of chronic insomniacs: a preliminary study. *Biological Psychiatry* 30:371–376.

Morrey et al. 1994. Activation of human monocytes by the pineal hormone melatonin. *Journal of Immunology* 153:2671–80.

Sandyk et al. 1992. Is postmenopausal osteoporosis related to pineal gland functions? *Internat J Neurosci* 62:215–25.

Zhdanova et al. 2001. Melatonin promotes sleep-like state in zebrafish. *Brain Res* 8:903(1–2):263–8.

Mushrooms (Immune-Boosting Varieties)

Definition: Some species of mushrooms and yeast contain powerful compounds that boost immune defenses. Beta-D-glucan or beta 1, 3-D-glucan is the most important of these. Shiitake and maitake mushrooms, as well as yeast-containing herbs like *Cordyceps sinensis* and aloe vera contain beta-glucans. A beta-glucan compound called grifolin from maitake and lentinan from shiitake, have been the subject of several scientific inquiries.

Scientific Updates: Beta-glucan has proven itself as powerful activator of white blood cells (macrophages), which attack and destroy invading microorganisms. Macrophages also produce cytokines that direct other immune functions and stimulate the production of more immune cells. Studied for decades, beta-glucan binds to white blood cells, triggering a reaction that boosts overall immunity. It also stimulates the production of interleukin-1, which activates T-lymphocytes. Beta-glucan also fights tumors by increasing certainly chemicals that destroy them. Studies show that people taking beta-glucan after surgery had less infection. It has also shown powerful antibacterial actions even with antibiotic-resistant varieties of bacteria. Beta-glucans also fight viruses and keep infections from spreading. Beta-glucans may also lower cholesterol and help regulate blood sugar.

Safety: There is no known toxicity or side effects from using beta-glucan, though it has not been subject to long term studies; and its safety in pregnant or nursing women has not been established. Don't use yeast products if you have a yeast allergy or yeast infection or are allergic to any molds. If you have an autoimmune disease, check with your doctor before using beta-glucans.

Product Forms: Beta-glucan can be isolated from baker's yeast and is sold as individual supplements or is often contained in products offering shiitake and maitake mushrooms and cordyceps.

Comments: You can buy dried shiitake mushrooms and use them in various dishes. Mushroom extracts are often combined with herbs like echinacea and garlic in immune-boosting combinations.

References

Beauvais et al. 2001. Glucan synthase complex of Aspergillus fumigatus. *J Bacteriol* 183(7):2273–9.

Behall et al. 1997. Effect of beta-glucan level in oar fiber extracts on blood lipids in men and women. *J Am Coll Nutr* 16(1)46–51.

Di Renzo et al. 1991. The function of human NK cells is enhanced by beta-glucan, a ligand of CR3 (CD11b/CS18). *Eur J Immunol* 21(7)1755–8.

Kenler et al. 1994. A phase II multiple center, double-blind, randomized, placebo-controlled study of three dosages of an immunomodulator (PGG-glucan) in high risk surgical patients. *Arch Surg* 129(11):1204–10.

Kulicke et al. 1997. Correlation between immunological activity, molecular mass and molecular structure of different (1-3)-beta-D-glucans. *Carbohydr Res* 297(2)135–42.

Liang et al. 1998. Enhanced clearance of a multiple antibiotic resistant Staphylococcus aureus in rats treated with PBB-glucan is associated with increased leukocyte counts and increased nedutrophil oxidative burst activity. *Int J Immunopharmacol* 20(11)595–614.

Patchen et al. 1998. Mobilization of peripheral progenitor cells by Betafectin PGG-glucan alone and in combination with granulocyte colony-stimulating factor. *Stem Cells* 16(3):208–17.

Penna, C., P.A. Dean, and H. Nelson. 1996. Pulmonary metastases neutralization and tumor rejection by in vivo administration of beta-glucan and bispecific antibody. *Int J Cancer* 65(3)377–82.

Sakurai et al. 1992. Enhancement of murine alveolar macrophage functions by orally administered beta-glucan. *Int J Immunopharmacol* 14(5)821–30.

Thornton, B. et al. 1996. Analysis of the sugar specificity and molecular location of the beta-glucan binding lectin site of complement receptor type 3. *J Immunol* 156(3):1235–46.

Tsiapali et al. 2001. Glucans exhibit weak antioxidant activity, but stimulate macrophage free radical activity. *Free Radic Biol Med* 15:30(4):393–402.

NADH

Definition: NADH, (nicotinamide adenine dinucleotide) is a vital co-factor that makes enzymatic reactions possible throughout the body. NADH is essential in the production of energy and contributes to the production of L-dopa, which is converted into a neurotransmitter called dopamine.

Recommended for: Alzheimer's disease, Parkinson's disease, jet lag, chronic fatigue syndrome, depression, athletic endurance, high cholesterol

Scientific Updates: Studies support the use of NADH for everything from jet lag to athletic stamina. Scientist also believe supplemental NADH can benefit Alzheimer's disease, chronic fatigue syndrome, Parkinson's disease and depression. In one trial, it appeared to enhance alertness and mental sharpness in test subjects who were subject to time zone changes. These benefits may be due to NADH's ability to boost blow flow and energy metabolism in the brain.

Safety: NADH appears to be safe when doses do not exceed 5 mg daily. There are no studies on its safety for children, pregnant or nursing women, or those with severe liver or kidney disease.

Product Forms: NADH is available in tablet or capsule form is sometimes added to athletic formulas or meal replacements.

Comments: The typical dosage for supplemental NADH ranges from 5 to 50 mg daily.

References

Birkmayer et al. 1993. Nicotinamide adenine dinucleotide (NADH)–a new therapeutic approach to Parkinson's disease. Comparison of oral and parenteral application. *Acta Neurol Scand Suppl* 146:32–35.

Birkmayer et al. 1991. The coenzyme nicotinamide adenine dinucleotide (NADH) as biological antidepressive agent: experience with 205 patients. *New Trends Clin Neuropharmacology* 5:19–25.

Birkmayer, J. 1996. Coenzyme nicotinamide adenine dinucleotide: new therapeutic approach for improving dementia of the Alzheimer type. *Ann Clin Lab Sci* 26:1–9.

Forsyth et al. 1999. Therapeutic effects of oral NADH on the symptoms of patients with chronic fatigue syndrome. *Ann Allergy Asthma Immunol* 82:185–191.

Ido et al. 2001. NADH: sensor of blood flow need in brain, muscle, and other tissues. *FASEB J* 15(8):1419–21.

Kay et al. 2000. Stabilized NADH as a countermeasure for jet lag. Presented at: 48th International Congress of Aviation and Space Medicine; September 17–21, Rio de Janeiro, Brazil.

Natural Progesterone

Definition: The idea of obtaining natural progesterone from wild yam has generated a great deal of controversy and misinformation. It has been thought by some that a woman's body can covert diosgenin from wild yam root into progesterone, which is not accurate. Wild yam does contain phytoestrogens, which may be a benefit for several female complaints. Moreover, the structure of diosgenin is close to that of progesterone, but according to current opinion, science does not support its automatic conversion to progesterone in the body. There are natural progesterone products, which are often added to wild yam cream that are synthesized from soy or from the diosgenin in wild yam.

Recommended for: PMS, heavy periods, cramping, fibroids, fibrocystic breast disease, menopause, osteoporosis, anovulatory cycles, dysfunctional uterine bleeding, endometriosis

Scientific Updates: Currently natural progesterone cream has only been studied by John Lee, M.D., who is convinced that taking progesterone through the skin greatly benefits women for several disorders: PMS, fibroids, fibrocystic breast disease, menopause and osteoporosis. One of his limited studies uses a 3 percent progesterone cream that showed an increase in bone density and reduction in fractures. New micronization processes make it possible now to take progesterone synthesized from natural sources orally. Although we need more studies on topical progesterone, new evidence does suggest that natural progesterone can prevent uterine tissue abnormalities, prevent bone loss and may also protect the heart. A recent study confirms that natural progesterone is absorbed from the skin into the saliva.

Safety: Anyone taking other hormones should check with their doctor before taking natural progesterone. Pregnant or nursing women should not take it, and women who have hormonally driven cancers such as breast or uterine should not take natural progesterone without their doctor's consent and supervision.

Product Forms: Topical natural progesterone products come in creams, gels, ointments and tinctures. Oral forms include capsules, teas and sublingual tablets. Keep in mind that without the micronization process, oral progesterone is poorly absorbed. USP progesterone made from soybeans can be considered natural, unlike progestins used in oral contraceptives. Norethindrone is not actually progesterone but is close in structure and functions the same for some women.

Comments: It is important to understand that diosgenin is extracted from the Mexican wild yam in the laboratory and is then converted to pregnenolone and then progesterone. We know now that female body cannot convert diosgenin to progesterone. Products that contain more than 400 mg of progesterone per ounce of cream usually need a prescription. A product that contains less than 15 mg of progesterone per ounce of cream will have little value. Use most products at half a teaspoon twice daily, and rotate sites of applications from time to time. To be effective, look for products that contain 400 mg of progesterone per ounce.

References

Abdalla et al. 1985. Prevention of bone mineral loss in postmenopausal women by norethisterone. *Obstet Gynecol* 66:789–92.

Kim et al. 1996. Antiproliferative effects of low-dose micronized progesterone. *Fertility and Sterility* 65(2):323–331.

Lee J. 1990. Osteoporosis Reversal, The Role of Progesterone. *International Clinical Nutrition Review* 10(3):384–391.

O'Leary et al. 2000. Salivary, but not serum or urinary levels of progesterone are elevated after topical application of progesterone cream to pre- and post-menopausal women. Clin Endocrinol (Oxf). 53(5):615–20.

Riis et al. 1987. The effect of percutaneous estradiol and natural progesterone on postmenopausal bone loss. *American J Ob/Gynecology* 156:61–65.

Zaffaroni et al. 1997 .Topical progesterone as support for the luteal phase in induced cycles. *Minerva Ginecol* 49(7–8):361–4.

Phosphatidylserine

Definition: Phosphatidylserine (PS) is a phospholipid that comprises cell membranes. It is abundantly found in the brain and may work to protect and even to enhance mental function. PS is found in trace amounts in the diets, and tiny amounts are present in lecithin. The body manufactures PS from other phospholipids. Supplements are derived from both bovine and soy sources. Scientists believe some older individuals may not synthesize enough PS; they also believe this deficiency is related to memory deficits.

Recommended for: early Alzheimer's disease, depression, senile dementia, age-related memory impairment, behavioral disorders, ADHD, learning disorders, Parkinson's disease

Scientific Updates: Studies have found that taking PS at 300 mg per day for three to six months resulted in memory improvement in test groups of older individuals and in those with early Alzheimer's disease. In one double-blind study, mental improvement was up almost 16 percent and continued for weeks after supplementation ceased. Other studies confirm that PS affects brain function. PS is not a cure for Alzheimer's disease but may slow its progression. The sooner you treat Alzheimer's the better. PS supplementation has also been shown to reverse amnesia in laboratory test animals. It may also benefit people with Parkinson's disease.

Safety: No significant side effects associated with PS have been consistently reported. At the time of writing, there were no well-known drug interactions with phosphatidylserine. Bovine sources of PS were thought to pose the threat of infection, so they have been replaced with soy-based PS.

Product Forms:. Soy-based PS supplements have replaced bovine products. There have been limited studies on the soy form.

Comments: Positive effects on mental function have been achieved using 200 to 500 mg per day of PS. Because most data was collected using bovine PS, it is not known if soy-based PS will perform the same way.

References

Crook et al. 1991. Effects of phosphatidylserine in age-associated memory impairment. *Neurology* 41:644–49.

Crook et al. 1992. Effects of phosphatidylserine in Alzheimer's disease. *Psychopharmacol Bull* 28:61–66.

Fünfgeld et al. 1989. Double-blind study with phosphatidylserine (PS) in Parkinsonian patients with senile dementia of Alzheimer's type. *Prog Clin Biol Res* 317:1235–46.

Furushiro et al. 1997. Effects of oral administration of soybean lecithin transphosphatidylated phosphatidylserine on impaired learning of passive avoidance in mice. *Jpn J Pharmacol* 75:447–50.

Maggioni et al. 1990. Effects of phosphatidylserine therapy in geriatric patients with depressive disorders. *Acta Psychiatr Scand* 81:265–70.

Schreiber et al. 2000. An open trial of plant-source derived phosphatydilserine for treatment of age-related cognitive decline. *Isr J Psychiatry Relat Sci* 37(4):302–7.

Suzuki et al. 2000. Effect of intracerebroventricular administration of soybean lecithin transphosphatidylated phosphatidylserine on scopolamine-induced amnesic mice. *Jpn J Pharmacol* 84(1):86–8.

Ulmann et al. 2001. Brain and hippocampus fatty acid composition in phospholipid classes of aged-relative cognitive deficit rats. *Prostaglandins Leukot Essent Fatty Acids* 64(3):189–95.

Pregnenolone

Definition: Pregnelonone is a hormone that is synthesized from cholesterol in several organs. Pregnenolone is a precursor to DHEA (dehydroepiandrosterone) and to progesterone. It has been called the master steroid in that it provides the building blocks for crucial hormones in the body. Pregnenolone exists as both free pregnenolone and as pregnenolone-sulfate. Its exact actions on body systems remain unclear.

Recommended for: enhanced brain function, memory deficiencies, Alzheimer's, mood disorders, chronic fatigue, cholesterol levels, lupus, immune weakness, multiple sclerosis, PMS, prostate disease, psoriasis, rheumatoid arthritis, gout, scleroderma, stress, spinal cord trauma

Scientific Updates: Several studies confirm pregnenolone's potent memory enhancing actions. It has also been found to improve sleep quality and to lessen periods of wakefulness. Pregnenolone may also help to negate the negative effects of stress by counteracting adrenal gland hormonal output that results in both mental and physical fatigue. It apparently acts to excite certain neurons in the brain that contribute to better focus, memory and mental performance. A link between low pregnenolone levels and depression has been made; and in cream form, pregnenolone was able to temporarily improve wrinkling. It has also been used for arthritic conditions and appears to improve joint mobility and pain. This anti-inflammatory effect may also benefit gout, lupus, scleroderma and psoriasis.

Safety: Because your body converts pregnenolone to DHEA, androgens and estrogens, don't use it without your physician's approval. Although studies have found the compound to be nontoxic, pregnenolone has not been subject to intensified long-term investigation. Because it also converts to aldosterone, blood pressure could rise when taking pregnenolone; therefore, anyone suffering from hypertension should not use it. High doses of pregnenolone could suppress immune function and may cause seizures in people with epilepsy. Pregnenolone may inhibit drugs used to treat epilepsy and depression. It may also raise progesterone levels and other hormones causing changes in the menstrual cycle, or interacting with hormone therapy such as birth control pills. It may also stimulate hormonally driven cancer of the breast, prostate, etc. The side effects and interactions of pregnenolone with other therapies are currently unknown. The effects of pregnenolone on pregnant or nursing women have not been established.

Product Forms: Stores sell pregnenolone in capsule form. Take this supplement as directed. Pregnenolone is also added to formulas designed to treat inflammatory diseases or to enhance mental performance.

Comments: Pregnenolone is generally sold in individual dosages ranging from 10 to 30 mg. Appropriate oral dosage amounts remain unknown as testing was done with injections. There is some speculation that starting with a low dose, then going to a higher, then subsequent lower dose may be more effective, but exact dosage amounts are unknown.

References

Ceccon et al. 2001. Distinct effect of pregnenolone sulfate on NMDA receptor subtypes. *Neuropharmacology* 40(4):491–500.

Flood et al. 1992. Memory-enhancing effects in male mice of pregnenolone and steroids metabolically derived from it. *Proc Natl Acad Sci* 9:1567–71.

George et al. 1994. CSF neuroactive steroids in affective disorders: pregnenolone, progesterone and DBI. *Biol Psychiatry* 35(10):775–80.

Grigoryev et al. 2000. Pregnenolone stimulates LNCaP prostate cancer cell growth via the mutated androgen receptor. *J Steroid Biochem Mol Biol* 1:5(1):1–10.

Gursoy et al. 2001. Pregnenolone protects mouse hippocampal (HT-22) cells against glutamate and amyloid beta protein toxicity. *Neurochem Res* 26(1):15–21.

Guth et al. 1994. Key role for pregnenolone in combination therapy that promotes recovery after spinal cord injury. 91:12308–312.

McGavack, T. 1951. The use of D 5-pregnenolone in various clinical disorders. *J Clin Endocrinol* 11(6):559–77.

Steiger et al. 1993. Neurosteroid pregnenolone induces sleep-EEG changes in man compatible with inverse agonistic GABAA-receptor modulation. *Brain Res* 615:267–74.

Sternberg, T. 1961. The hydrating effects of pregnenolone acetate on the human skin. *Curr Ther Res* (11):469–71.

Probiotics *(Acidophilus spp., Lactobacillus spp.)*

Definition: Certain substances that are soured such as active culture yogurt, buttermilk, certain cheeses, etc., contain *Lactobacillus acidophilus*, which enhances digestion and elimination. Acidophilus also helps to detoxify harmful bacteria by helping to restore "friendly bacteria," which keep certain microorganisms in check. Good food sources of acidophilus include the following: fermented milk products, including yogurt and kefir. High temperatures destroy acidophilus, so fermented milk products are not good sources if they've been warmed. Nondairy sources of acidophilus are available. All sources, whether liquid or capsule, should be refrigerated and taken on an empty stomach in the morning. Check expiration dates before purchasing any acidophilus product.

Recommended for: vaginal yeast infections, urinary tract infections, lactose intolerance, diarrhea, fibromyalgia, irritable bowel syndrome, lupus, high cholesterol, osteoporosis, indigestion, constipation, gas, post antibiotic therapy

Scientific Updates: Several studies show that acidophilus supplementation of women with recurring yeast infections decreased their infection rate by almost 75 percent after six months of treatment. *Lactobacillus acidophilus* has an impressive track record for the prevention and treatment of diarrhea and other gastrointestinal disorders. It may also lower cholesterol levels, prevent colon cancer, inhibit allergic responses and treat skin disorders and rashes. It also helps to put more calcium in the bones. New studies suggest that children who have been on antibiotic therapy can develop deranged intestinal flora, which may contribute to undetected yeast infections that can lead to disorders like ADHD.

Safety: Acidophilus is considered safe; however, anyone suffering from an allergy to milk products should use nondairy acidophilus products. If you have any serious gastrointestinal problems that require medical attention, check with your doctor before taking. Amounts exceeding ten billion viable *L. acidophilus* organisms daily may cause mild gastrointestinal distress.

Comments: Take acidophilus supplements after antibiotic therapy or their effects will be neutralized. Capsule, tablet, liquid or edible forms such as buttermilk, yogurt, etc., supply bacteria. Always check for expiration date, and use guaranteed bacterial count products with lacto and bifido bacteria (a minimum of one billion organisms per capsule). Keep the supplement refrigerated and away from heat or light. Enteric-coated capsules may be preferable for severe symptoms. Fructo-oligosaccharides are sometimes added to supplements for enhanced activity. Take probiotic supplements with food. Give infants or children who have been on antibiotic therapy a liquid acidophilus supplement for three months.

References

De Simone et al. 1993. The Role of Probiotics in Modulation of the Immune System in Man and in Animals. *Int J Immunother* 9:23–8.

Hilton et al. 1992. Ingestion of Yogurt Containing Lactobacillus Acidophilus as Prophylaxis for Candidal Vaginitis. *Ann Int Med* 116:353–7.

Isolauri et al. 2001. Probiotics in human disease. *Am J Clin Nutr* 73(6 Part 2):1142S–6S.

Isolauri, E. 2001. Probiotics in the prevention and treatment of allergic disease. *Pediatr Allergy Immunol* 12(S14):56–9.

Kawase, K. 1982. Effects of Nutrients on the Intestinal Microflora of Infants. *Jpn J Dairy Food Sci* 31:A241–A243.

Loizeau, E. 1993. Can Antibiotic-associated Diarrhea be Prevented? *Annales de Gastroenterologie et d Hepatologie* 29(1):15–8.

Lu, L. and W. Walker. 2001. Pathologic and physiological interactions of bacteria with the gastrointestinal epithelium. *Am J Clin Nutr* 73(6 Part 2):1124S–30S.

Saavedra, J. 2001. Clinical applications of probiotic agents. *Am J Clin Nutr* 73(6 Part 2):1147S–51S.

Wanke, C. 2001. Do probiotics prevent childhood illnesses? They show promise, but bigger studies are needed. *British Medical Journal* 2:322(7298):1318–9.

Proanthocyanidins

Definition: Also known as grape seed extract and pine bark extract, these oligomeric proanthocyanidins (OPCs) and procyanidolic oligomers made pycnogenol a household name. Proanthocyanidins are compounds that are members of the bioflavonoid family of nutrients. They have potent antioxidant actions, can help to preserve collagen and elastin in the skin and other tissues, and can reduce inflammation and swelling. Proanthocyanidins can be found most abundantly in pine bark, grape seed and grape skin.

Recommended for: visual problems, night blindness, venous insufficiency, allergies, joint disorders, blood vessel disorders, varicose veins, radiation exposure, diabetes, liver disorders, post-operative swelling

Scientific Updates: Proanthocyanidins have been shown to strengthen capillaries in as low a dose as 50 mg daily. They also help to improve chronic venous insufficiency at higher doses and can also improve vision. Proanthocyanidins have a better-than-usual ability to scavenge for dangerous free radicals, making them a more potent antioxidant the vitamin C or vitamin E. Other studies have shown that these flavonoids also protect against radiation and support the liver and may stop the abnormal reproduction of cells that form tumors.

Safety: Flavonoids in general are considered nontoxic and free of side effects. We excrete excess amounts of these nutrients, like vitamin C, in the urine. Currently, there were no well-known drug interactions with proanthocyanidins.

Product Forms: Proanthocyanidins may come under the name "pycnogenol" or other designated titles. You can purchase them as single supplements or in combination with other nutrients, in herbal extracts, capsules and tablets in antioxidant or anti-inflammatory formulas.

Comments: Taking 50 to 100 mg of proanthocyanidins daily is considered an average dose, although some practitioners like to start with a high saturating dose for a serious condition and then lower the dose. Optimal levels remain unknown. Taking proanthocyanidins may also enhance the action or preservation of vitamin C.

References

Baroch, J. 1984. Effect of Endotelon in postoperative edema. Results of a double-blind study versus placebo in 32 female patients. *Ann Chir Polast Esthet* 29:393–95.

Castillo et al. 2000. Antioxidant activity and radioprotective effects against chromosomal damage induced in vivo by X-rays of flavan-3-ols (Procyanidins) from grape seeds (Vitis vinifera): comparative study versus other phenolic and organic compounds. *J Agric Food Chem* 48(5):1738–45.

Corbe et al. 1988. Light vision and chorioretinal circulation. Study of the effect of procyanidalic oligomers. J Fr Ophtalmol 11:453–60.

Gusak et al. 2000. Application of preparation endotelon in complex treatment of chronic arterial insufficiency of lower extremities. *Klin Khir* (10):7–9.

Liviero, L. and E. Puglisis. 1994. Antimutagenic activity of procyanidins from vitis vinfera. *Fitother* 65:203–209.

Maffei et al. 1994. Free radical scavenging action and antienzyme activities of procyanidines from Vitis vinifera. A mechanism for their capillary protective action. *Arzn Forsch* 44:592–601.

Mitcheva et al. 1993. Biochemical and morphological studies on the effects of anthocyans and vitamin E on carbon tetrachloride induced liver injury. *Cell Mol Bio* 39(4):443–48.

Moini et al. 2000. Molecular aspects of procyanidin biological activity: disease preventative and therapeutic potentials. *Drug Metabol Drug Interact* 17(1–4):237–59.

Moini et al. 2000. Enzyme inhibition and protein-binding action of the procyanidin-rich french maritime pine bark extract, pycnogenol: effect on xanthine oxidase. *J Agric Food Chem* 48(11):5630–9.

Pyruvate (*Sodium Pyruvate, Calcium Pyruvate, Potassium Pyruvate, Magnesium Pyruvate, Dihydroxyacetone Pyruvate [DHAP]*)

Definition: Pyruvate (in the form pyruvic acid) is a natural substance created in the body when carbohydrates and protein are broken down. It is also found in red apples, cheese, dark beer and red wine. Current interest centers on its purported ability to stimulate weight loss and to contribute to the formation of lean muscle mass.

Recommended for: weight loss, obesity, muscle building, athletic stamina and performance, insulin resistance

Scientific Updates: Pyruvate may work to boost weight loss by increasing the resting metabolic rate and by reducing body fat at a faster pace. Other studies suggest that pyruvate supplements may improve exercise endurance and stamina. Preliminary research also shows that pyruvate gathers dangerous free radicals, and due to its strong antioxidant effect, may inhibit the growth of cancerous tumors. It may also reduce cholesterol levels and insulin resistance and boost the ability of heart muscle to recover faster after periods of stress.

Safety: High intake of pyruvate can cause stomach upset, gas, bloating and diarrhea. Currently, there are no well-known drug interactions with pyruvate. Its effect on pregnan/nursing women remains unknown.

Product Forms: Pyruvate is added to weight-loss powders and other supplements. Because you need such large doses, it may be more practical to buy it as a single supplement in powdered form. In addition, because you require so much pyruvate to achieve desired results, make sure your source is pure and uncontaminated.

Comments: Human trials have used a minimum of 30 grams of pyruvate per day (a considerable amount). Lower doses may not create any effects. Many weight-loss supplements only contain very small amounts of pyruvate, which will probably offer little to no benefit.

References

Deboer et al. 1993. Pyruvate enhances recovery of rat hearts after ischemia and reperfusion by preventing free radical generation. *Am J Physiol* 265:H1571–76.

Ivy et al. 1994. Effects of pyruvate on the metabolism and insulin resistance of obese Zucker rats. *Am J Clin Nutr* 59:331–37.

Stanko et al. 1994. Pyruvate supplementation of a low-cholesterol, low-fat diet: Effects on plasma lipid concentration and body composition in hyperlipidemic patients. *Am J Clin Nutr* 59:423–27.

Stanko et al. 1994. Pyruvate inhibits growth of mammary adenocarcinoma 13762 in rats. *Cancer Res* 54:1004–1007.

Stanko et al. 1992. Body composition, energy utilization, and nitrogen metabolism with a 4.25-MJ/d low-energy diet supplemented with pyruvate. *Am J Clin Nutr* 56(4):630–5.

Stanko et al. 1990. Enhanced leg exercise endurance with a high-carbohydrate diet and dihyroxyacetone and pyruvate. *J Appl Phys* 69(5):1651–56.

Sukala, W. 1998. Pyruvate: beyond the marketing hype. *Int J Sport Nutr* 8(3):241–9.

Vinpocetine

Definition: Vinpocetine, (ethyl apovincaminate) is synthesized from vincamine, an alkaloid found in the periwinkle plant (a common purple-flowered ground cover). Ongoing research on vinca alkaloid components has shown that it boosts blood flow to brain tissue thereby improving the brain's supply of oxygen and glucose. This effect protects brain cells from oxygen deprivation and can enhance mental performance. Unlike prescription drugs, vinpocetine has comparable actions with far fewer side effects.

Recommended for: strokes, senile dementia, Alzheimer's disease, cerebral circulatory disorders, altitude sickness (prevention also), memory deficits, situations where the brain's oxygen supply is temporarily cut off, tinnitus and eye disorders due to blocked circulation, incontinence

Special Instructions: Several studies back the ability of vinpocetine to protect brain cells from oxygen deprivation in cases of atherosclerosis. It also appears to do the same after ministrokes or other situations where the brain's oxygen supply is interrupted. By boosting blood supply through vessel dilation, vinpocetine provides the brain more glucose and ATP. ATP provides cells with energy. This triple effect prevents brain cell death, which can cause impaired mental capacity. Numerous clinical studies show that vinpocetine reduces resistance in blood vessels and actually widens them, which also discourages the formation of clots. It is also able to stimulate noradrenergic neurons in the brain which enhances mental functions and the speed in which information is processed that often declines with age. It has also shown the ability to prevent or lessen altitude sickness due to oxygen deprivation at high altitudes and may benefit tinnitus and retinal disease due to compromised circulation. One unexpected application is for urge incontinence and bladder control.

Safety: Vinpocetine technically is not a "natural" compound and should be taken only under the advisement of your health care practitioner. No serious side effects have been reported in any of the clinical trials. It should not be taken with Coumadin (warfarin) because it may lessen the potency of these blood thinning drugs. One report of the loss of certain white blood cells has been associated with vinpocetine supplementation. Safety in pregnant or nursing women, young children, or those with severe liver or kidney disease has not been established.

Product Forms: Vinpocetine usually comes in 10 mg capsules. It is best to take it with meals for optimal absorption.

Comments: The usual dose of vinpocetine is between 5 and 10 mg taken two to three times daily, but even doses half that size can be effective. Be aware that if you suffer from cerebral vascular disorders, it may take several weeks of vinpocetine therapy to see any improvement.

References

Bereczki et al. 1999. A systematic review of vinpocetine therapy in acute ischaemic stroke. *Eur J Clin Pharmacol* 55:349–352.

Gulyas et al. 2001. The effect of a single-dose intravenous vinpocetine on brain metabolism in patients with ischemic stroke. *Orv Hetil* 4:142(9):443–9.

Hitzenberger et al. 1990. Influence of vinpocetine on warfarin-induced inhibition of coagulation. *Int J Clin Pharmacol Ther Toxicol* 28:323–328.

Horvath, S. 2001. The use of vinpocetine in chronic disorders caused by cerebral hypoperfusion. *Orv Hetil* 25:142(8):383–9.

Lohmann et al. 1992. Bioavailability of vinpocetine and interference of the time of application with food intake. *Arzneimittelforschung* 42:914–917.

Truss et al 2000. Initial clinical experience with the selective phosphodiesterase-I isoenzyme inhibitor vinpocetine in the treatment of urge incontinence and low compliance bladder. *World J Urol* 18(6):439–43.

Index of Health Conditions

About the Author

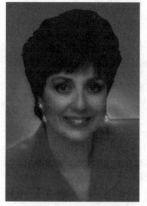

RITA ELKINS, M.H., has worked as an author and research specialist in the health field for the last ten years, and possesses a strong background in both conventional and alternative health therapies. She is the author of numerous books, including *The Complete Home Health Advisor,* which combines standard medical treatments with holistic alternatives for more than 100 diseases, *Solving the Depression Puzzle, The Complete Fiber Fact Book,* and *Soy Smart Health,* which recently won Health Book of the Year from *ForeWord Magazine.* Rita has also authored dozens of booklets exploring the documented value of natural supplements like SAMe, noni, blue-green algae, chitosan, stevia and many more. She received an honorary Master Herbalist Degree from the College of Holistic Health and Healing in 1994.

Rita is frequently consulted for the formulation of herbal blends and has recently joined the 4-Life Research Medical Advisory Board. She is a regular contributor to *Let's Live* and *Great Life* magazines and is a frequent host on radio talk shows exploring natural health topics. She lectures nationwide on the science behind natural compounds and collaborates with medical doctors on various projects. Rita's publications and lectures have been used by companies like Nature's Sunshine, 4-Life Research, Enrich, NuSkin, and Nutraceutical to support the credibility of natural and integrative health therapies.

Rita resides in Utah, is married, and has two daughters and two granddaughters.

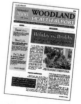